Stress Fractures

Stress Fractures

Peter Brukner
MBBS, DRCOG, FACSM, FACSP
Sports Physician and Clinic Director,
Olmpic Park Sports Medicine Centre, Melbourne

Kim Bennell
BAppSc (Phsio), PhD
Senior Lecturer, School of Physiotherapy,
University of Melbourne

Gordon Matheson
MD, PhD
Associate Professor of Functional Restoration and
Director of Sports Medicine
Stanford University School of Medicine, Stanford,
California

SETON HALL UNIVERSITY
UNIVERSITY LIBRARIES
SO. ORANGE, NJ 07079-2671

b
**Blackwell
Science**

© 1999 by Blackwell Science Asia Pty Ltd

First published 1999

Editorial offices:

54 University Street, Carlton
Victoria 3053, Australia

Osney Mead, Oxford OX2 0EL

25 John Street, London WC1N 2BL

23 Ainslie Place, Edinburgh EH3 6AJ

350 Main Street, Malden
MA 02148-5018, USA

Other editorial offices:

Blackwell Wissenschafts-Verlag GmbH
Kurfürstendamm 57
10707 Berlin, Germany

Zehetnergasse 6
1140 Wien, Austria

Edited by   Deborah Doyle
Typeset by Graphicraft Typesetters, Hong Kong
Design by The University of Melbourne
               Design and Print Centre
Printed in   Australia

Distributors

NORTH AMERICA

Human Kinetics
PO Box 5076
Champaign, IL 61825-5076

1-800-747-4457
e-mail: humank@hkusa.com

CANADA

Human Kinetics
475 Devonshire Road Unit 100
Windsor, ON N8Y 2L5

1-800-465-7301 (in Canada only)
e-mail: humank@hkcanada.com

EUROPE

Human Kinetics
PO Box 1W14, Leeds, LS16 6TR
United Kingdom

(44) 1132 781708
e-mail: humank@hkeurope.com

Australasia

Blackwell Science Asia Pty Ltd
54 University Street
Carlton, Victoria, 3053, Australia

Orders: Tel: 03 9347 0300
                 fax: 03 9347 5001
                 e-mail: info@blacksci-asia.com.au
internet: www.blackwell-science.com.au

CATALOGUING-IN-PUBLICATION DATA

Brukner, Peter.
Stress fractures

Includes index.
ISBN 0 86793 01 2

1. Stress fractures (Orthopedics). 2. Overuse injuries. I. Bennell, Kim. II. Matheson, Gordon Omar, 1952–. III. Title

Contents

Preface

In the quarter century since the landmark book about stress fractures by Michael Devas was published, considerable advances have been made in our understanding of stress fracture. During this period, the amount of training undertaken by most serious athletes has increased dramatically, and as a result there has been a concomitant increase in the number of overuse injuries in general and stress fractures in particular.

All three authors of this book have had a longstanding clinical and research interest in stress fractures, and have been published widely on the subject. The purpose of the book is to bring together the authors' and other people's research results in an organised way. We first cover the epidemiological and pathophysiological factors, risk factors, diagnosis and treatment of stress fractures, then move on to the various types of stress fracture, which we cover on a regional basis.

Writing the book would not have been possible without the help of many of our medical colleagues who have given us the benefit of their experience and expertise. Our biggest thank you goes to Winne Meeuwisse, who so diligently reviewed a number of the chapters. We also wish to thank the following colleagues, who reviewed sections of the manuscript: Jason Agosta, Chris Bradshaw, Doug Clement, Ken Crichton, Julian Feller, Jim Garrick, Stan Herring, Bill Kohl, Carol Macera, Lyle Micheli, Martin Schwellnus, Jack Taunton, Susan White, and Preston Wiley. We also wish to thank Jock Anderson, Steven Kiss and Chris Bradshaw, who helped us by providing many of the pictorial images. Without the secretarial support of Portia Leet and Deborah Horne, we would not have made it. We have also been fortunate in having the support of Shirley Green, Neil Dickson and Mark Robertson of our publisher Blackwell Science Asia, and Debbie Doyle, who was a patient and skillful editor.

Peter Brukner, Kim Bennell, Gordon Matheson

About the authors

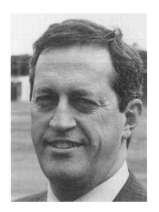

Peter Brukner is a sports physician and clinic director at Olympic Park Sports Medicine Centre in Melbourne, Australia. He is an inaugural Fellow of the Australian College of Sports Physicians, and an Honorary Fellow of both the American College of Sports Medicine and the Australian Sports Medicine Federation. He has served two terms as president of the Australian College of Sports Physicians, as well as a term as the college's chief examiner.

Peter has had extensive experience as a team physician for the Olympic Games, the Commonwealth Games, and world championships in a number of sports, and has been involved with professional Melbourne football teams. He is a former editor of *Sport Health* and is at present senior associate editor of the *Clinical Journal of Sport Medicine*. He has co-authored two books: *Food for Sport* (with Karen Inge) and *Clinical Sports Medicine* (with Karim Khan), as well as a number of chapters and original articles.

He has presented papers at conferences held in New Zealand, the Philippines, Japan, Germany, Greece, the Netherlands, South Africa, the United Kingdom, and the United States.

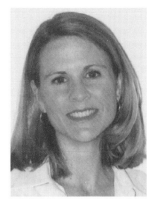

Kim Bennell is a senior lecturer in musculoskeletal physiotherapy at the School of Physiotherapy, The University of Melbourne, Australia, and is principal physiotherapist at Melbourne Fitness Club Physiotherapy. She is a committee member for both the Sports Physiotherapy Group and Sports Medicine Australia's Medicine and Science for Women in Sport Committee.

In 1996, Kim completed a PhD for which she investigated the effects of excercise on the skeletal system in which she especially focused on stress fractures in athletes. She has received a number of research grants, including one from the National Health and Medical Research Council in order to investigate the effects of excercise on the skeleton during growth.

In 1994, Kim won the annual Young Investigator Award at Sports Medicine Australia's International Conference in Science and Medicine in Sport, for her research into stress fractures. She has also won LaTrobe University's Graduate Research Prize for her research in the sports medicine area. Kim has been widely published in peer-reviewed scientific journals, and has been invited to speak about exercise and bone health at several national and international conferences.

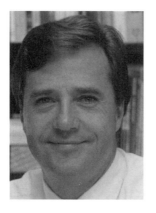

Gordon Matheson is associate professor and chief of the Division of Sports Medicine, Department of Functional Restoration, School of Medicine at Stanford University, California. He is also director of the Sports Medicine Program for Stanford's Department of Athletics. He is heading Stanford's new academic sports medicine initiative by developing clinical research and teaching components, and by working towards establishing an institute.

Gordon is editor-in-chief of the *Physician and Sportsmedicine* journal, is a past president of the Canadian Academy of Sport Medicine, and is founding editor-in-chief of the *Clinical Journal of Sport Medicine*. He has served as team physician to Canada's Olympic hockey team, and to the Vancouver Canucks team in the National Hockey League. He has received research grants from the Alberta Heritage Foundation for Medical Research, the Medical Research Council of Canada, the Natural Sciences and Engineering Research Council, and the British Columbia Health Research Foundation.

Introduction

Physical exercise has beneficial effects on a number of physiologic systems, including the skeleton. However, combined with potential risk factors, unwise training practises may harm these systems. A stress fracture represents one form of breakdown in the skeletal system.[1]

Definition of a stress fracture

A stress fracture can be defined as a partial or complete bone fracture that results from repeated application of a stress lower than the stress required in order to fracture the bone in a single loading.[2]

A historical perspective

Stress fractures were first described in 1855 by Briethaupt,[3] a Prussian military physician, who observed foot pain and swelling in young military recruits unaccustomed to the rigors of basic training. He considered this to be an inflammatory reaction in the tendon sheaths as a result of trauma, and he called the condition *Fussgeschwulst*. In 1887, Pauzat[4] suspected that the periosteum was involved in the condition, but it was not until the advent of radiographs that the signs and symptoms could be attributed to fractures in the metatarsals.[5] The condition then became known as a 'march fracture' because there was a close association between marching and the onset of symptoms. Stress fractures were first noticed in civilians in 1921 by Deutschlander,[6] who reported six cases in women. However, it was not until 1956 – more than a century after they had been identified in military recruits – that they were recognized in athletes.[7]

A variety of terms have been used to describe stress fractures, for varying periods. The terms include 'march fracture', 'Deutschlander's fracture', 'pied force', 'fatigue fracture', 'crack fracture', 'spontaneous fracture', 'insufficiency fracture', 'pseudofracture' and 'exhaustion fracture'.[6,8–12] Virtually all the terms have been intended to describe some etiologic attribute of the stress injuries of bone. In recent years, the most commonly used term has been 'stress fracture'.

Following radiographic description of metatarsal stress fractures, many and varied theories were set out in order to explain the injury's etiology. Most of the reports were based on series that were small, and the theories proposed involved mechanical factors such as spasticity and spasm of the interossei,[6,13,14] flat forefoot,[14] or inflammatory reactions such as nonsuppurative osteomyelitis.[9,10] Other theories included nutritional deficit,[15] polyhypovitaminosis,[15] and local periostitis secondary to hematogenous sepsis.[6] The current theories of stress-fracture development are discussed in Chapter 1.

Overuse injuries

Stress fractures represent overuse injuries of bone. In sports medicine, overuse injuries have been increasing as a problem over the past two decades. This has been because of a trend towards increased volume of training in all sports. An overuse injury occurs when repetitive microtrauma overloads a tissue's capacity to repair itself.

Overuse injuries present the practitioner with a number of challenges: first, to determine the diagnosis; second, to determine the treatment; and third, and most difficult, to determine why the overuse injury has occurred and to take steps to ensure it does not recur.

A cause has to be found for every overuse injury. The cause may be evident immediately, such as doubling of training quantity, poor footwear or an obvious biomechanical abnormality, or it may be more subtle, such as running on a cambered surface, muscle imbalance, or leg-length discrepancy. The causes of overuse injuries are usually divided into extrinsic factors, such as training, surfaces, shoes, equipment, and environmental conditions, or into intrinsic factors, such as malalignment, leg-length discrepancy, muscle imbalance, muscle weakness, lack of flexibility, and body composition. The factors that are possibly involved in development of overuse injuries are set out in Table A. Risk factors for stress fractures are specifically discussed in Chapter 3.

In the first two chapters, the pathophysiology and epidemiology of stress fractures are covered. In chapters 4 and 5, a general overview of diagnosis and treatment of stress fractures is provided, and in the subsequent chapters, management of specific stress fractures is described in detail on a regional basis.

Table A Overuse injuries: predisposing factors

Extrinsic factors	Intrinsic factors
Training errors	Malalignment
Excessive volume	Pes planus
Excessive intensity	Pes cavus
Rapid increase	Rearfoot varus
Sudden change	Tibia vara
Excessive fatigue	Genu valgum
Inadequate recovery	Genu varum
Faulty technique	Patella alta
Surfaces	Femoral neck
Hard	anteversion
Soft	Tibial torsion
Cambered	Leg-length discrepancy
Shoes	Muscle imbalance
Inappropriate	Muscle weakness
Worn out	Lack of flexibility
Equipment	Generalized muscle
Inappropriate	tightness
Environmental	Focal areas of
conditions	muscle thickening
Hot	Restricted joint
Cold	range of motion
Humid	Sex, size, and body
Psychological factors	composition
Inadequate nutrition	

Source: Adapted and reproduced, with permission, from Brukner P and Khan K, Clinical Sports Medicine. *Sydney: McGraw-Hill, 1993: 17 (table 2.2).*

References

[1] Grimston SK, Zernicke RF. Exercise-related stress responses in bone. *Journal of Applied Biomechanics* 1993; 9: 2–14.

[2] Martin AD, McCulloch RG. Bone dynamics: stress, strain and fracture. *Journal of Sports Sciences* 1987; 5: 155–163.

[3] Briethaupt MD. Fur pathologie des menschlichen fusses. *Medizinische Zeitung* 1855; 24: 169–177.

[4] Pauzat. De la periostite osteoplastique des metatarsiens a la suite de la marche. *Achives de Medecin et Pharmacie Militaire* 1887; 337.

[5] Stechow AW. Fussoedem und roentgenstrahlen. *Deutsch Mil-Aerztl Zeitung* 1897; 26: 465–471.

[6] Deutschlander C. Ueber eine eigenartige mittelfuszerkrankung. *Zentralbl. f. Chir* 1921; 48: 1422–1426.

[7] Devas MB, Sweetnam R. Stress fractures of the fibula: a review of 50 cases in athletes. *Journal of Bone and Joint Surgery* 1956; 38B: 818–829.

[8] Dodd H. Pied force or march foot. *British Journal of Surgery* 1933; 21: 131–144.

[9] Roberts SM, Vogt EC. Pseudofracture of the tibia. *Journal of Bone and Joint Surgery* 1939; 21: 891–898.

10 Weaver JB, Francisco CB. Pseudofractures: a manifestation of non-suppurative osteomyelitis. *Journal of Bone and Joint Surgery* 1940; 22: 610–615.

11 Burrows HJ. Fatigue fractures of the fibula. *Journal of Bone and Joint Surgery* 1948; 30B: 266–279.

12 Hullinger CW. Insufficiency fracture of the calcaneus: similar to march fracture of the metatarsal. *Journal of Bone and Joint Surgery* 1944; 26: 751–757.

13 Jansen M. March fractures. *Journal of Bone and Joint Surgery* 1926; 8: 262–267.

14 Sloane D, Sloane MF. March foot. *American Journal of Surgery* 1936; 31: 167–169.

15 Morris JM, Blickenstaff LD. *Fatigue Fractures: A Clinical Study*. Springfield, Illinois: Charles C. Thomas, 1967.

Chapter 1

The pathophysiology of stress fractures

*B*one is a specialized connective tissue that comprises organic material (mainly Type I collagen) and minerals (mainly calcium hydroxyapatite). Similar to other connective tissues of the musculoskeletal system, bone is able to adapt to repeated mechanical load by changing its microscopic and macroscopic architectural configuration. In order to best appreciate stress fractures' clinical manifestations, it is necessary to understand bone's basic biologic and mechanical responses to physical loading. In this chapter, bone structure and function are reviewed as they relate to the process of remodeling and to adaptation to physical loading.

Bone biology

BONE CELLS

Bone's biologic adaptability to repetitive strain is mediated by cells surrounded by a mineralized connective tissue matrix of collagen fibers and ground substance. Bone cells arise from various cell lines and perform various functions, including matrix formation, mineralization, and resorption. Osteoblasts are derived from local bone marrow mesenchymal cells and are located on all bone surfaces in which active bone formation is occurring.[1] Their main function is to synthesize and secrete bone's organic matrix. Once osteoblasts stop forming bone, they may either decrease their synthetic activity and remain on the bone's surface, whereby they are known as bone-lining cells, or surround themselves with matrix and become osteocytes. Compared with osteoblasts, bone-lining cells are elongated and contain fewer organelles. Their main role is to contract and secrete enzymes that remove the thin layer of osteoid that covers the mineralized matrix. Osteoclasts are thereby able to attach to bone and begin resorption.[2]

Osteocytes comprise more than 90% of the mature human skeleton's bone cells. They are connected to adjacent osteocytes, active osteoblasts and bone-lining cells by numerous cytoplasmic projections that travel in channels (canaliculi) through mineralized matrix.[3] These interconnections may enable the cells to sense bone deformation by mechanical loads and to coordinate the remodeling process.

Osteoclasts are derived from extraskeletal, hematopoietic stem cells. They are large, motile, multinucleated cells that are found on bone surfaces undergoing resorption. To resorb the bone matrix, osteoclasts bind to the bone surface and create an acidic environment by secreting protons and enzymes.[4]

EXTRACELLULAR MATRIX

Bone's extracellular matrix consists of both inorganic and organic components. The inorganic component contributes approximately 65% of bone's wet weight and consists of mainly calcium and phosphate in crystals of hydroxyapatite. Other ions within the bone matrix, in much smaller quantities, include carbonate, citrate, fluoride, magnesium and chloride. Bone's inorganic matrix performs two essential functions: it serves as an ion reservoir and gives bone most of its strength and stiffness. The organic components are collagen fibrils and an interfibrillar ground substance composed of as many as 200 noncollagenous proteins, including osteocalcin, osteonectin, osteopontin, and various glycoproteins. These organic constituents give bone its flexibility and resilience, and the matrix macromolecules seem to contribute to bone's structure and functional qualities. Most of the organic matrix is produced by osteoblasts, and the most abundant protein is Type I collagen. Collagen molecules are secreted into the extracellular space as procollagen. They are then assembled into fibrils that are arranged so spaces exist between molecules in order to accommodate the calcium and phosphate crystals.[2]

BONE STRUCTURE

The skeleton is composed of cortical and trabecular bone. Eighty percent of the skeleton comprises cortical bone, the densely compacted outer layer of all bones; the other 20% comprises trabecular (cancellous) bone, the meshwork of thin plates within the cortical shell. Both types of bone contribute to a given bone's strength, and individual bones contain varying proportions of each type. Appendicular, long bones are mainly cortical; the exception is at the metaphysis and epiphysis. The vertebral bodies and pelvic bones are largely trabecular. Compared with cortical bone, trabecular bone has greater porosity and is less able to withstand compressive forces. It also has a greater surface-to-volume ratio and a higher rate of metabolic activity, so it responds more rapidly to changes in mechanical loads.

Under light microscopy, it may be seen that cortical or trabecular bone consists of lamellar or woven bone. Lamellar bone is highly organized, densely packed collagen fibrils that are found in trabecular bone, on the inner and outer circumferential lamellae of cortical bone, on the interstitial lamellae of cortical bone, and in osteons or haversian systems. Osteons are the basic structural unit that more than two-thirds of adult cortical bone comprises. They consist of a series of concentric layers of mineralized matrix that surrounds a central lumen named the Haversian canal. This canal contains blood vessels and nerve fibers. Along each lamella's outer boundaries there are small cavities known as lacunae, and each lacuna houses one osteocyte. Numerous small canaliculi radiate from each lacuna in a network that connects the lacunae of adjacent lamellae and ultimately the Haversian canal. Osteons are separated from each other by cement lines that are thin layers of organic matrix. It is these cement lines that cracks in the bone matrix tend to follow.[2]

Woven bone is immature bone composed of irregularly arranged collagen fibers. It forms the embryonic skeleton and is then resorbed and replaced by mature bone as the skeleton develops. Although it is rarely present in the normal human skeleton after the person has reached four or five years of age, it can appear at any age in response to bone or soft-tissue injury, metabolic and neoplastic diseases, inflammation, or treatments that stimulate bone formation.

Bone loading

During physical activity, forces from ground impact and muscle contraction result in bone *stress*, which is defined as the load or force per unit area that develops on a plane surface, and in bone *strain*, which is defined as deformation of or change in bone dimension. In clinical terms, stress is a measure of the load applied, and strain is a measure of the amount of lengthening or deformation that occurs in a given direction.

When physical activity is undertaken, contact with the ground generates forces within the body. During running, vertical ground-reaction force (GRF) has been shown to vary from two to five times body weight,[5] and during jumping and landing activities, GRFs can reach 12 times body weight.[6] Transient impulse forces associated with GRFs are propagated upward from the foot and undergo attenuation as they pass toward the head.[7,8] A number of factors influence the impact forces' magnitude, propagation and attenuation. The factors include running speed, fatigue, type of foot strike, body weight, surface, terrain, and footwear.[9–11]

FACTORS THAT INFLUENCE BONE'S RESPONSE TO LOADING

These factors are listed in the following summary.

SUMMARY

> The main factors that influence bone's response to loading are
> - the load's direction
> - bone geometry
> - bone microarchitecture
> - bone density
> - muscle contraction.

Bone's stress–strain behavior is strongly dependent on the bone microstructure's orientation with reference to the direction of loading: a characteristic known as anisotropy. Although a complex relationship exists between loading patterns and mechanical properties, cortical bone is generally stronger and stiffer in the longitudinal direction than in the transverse direction. Trabecular bone is strongest along the lines of the trabeculae.[12]

Forces applied to bone can produce loading in tension, compression, bending, shear, and torsion (Fig. 1.1). In both the transverse and the longitudinal direction, human cortical bone withstands greater stress in compression than in tension, and greater stress in tension than in shear. With reference to bending, bone is subjected to a combination of tensile loads on one side and compressive loads on the other. Failure begins on the tensile side because adult bone is weaker in tension than in compression.[13] During activity, bone is subjected to a combination of loading modes. The loading patterns' complexity has been demonstrated in studies in which strains on the anteromedial surface of the human adult tibia during walking, running, and vigorous activity were measured.[14–17] During walking and running gait, development of strain on bone has been measured as a series of discrete events whereby bone is deformed from a particular direction, is released, and is then loaded from another direction. Stress values calculated from these measurements showed that compressive stresses predominated at heel strike, followed by high-tensile stresses at push-off (Fig. 1.2).[18]

A bone's geometry greatly influences the bone's strength. For tension and compression loads, a bone's strength is proportional to the bone cross-sectional area. A larger bone is therefore more resistant to fracture, because it distributes the internal forces over a larger surface area, and this results in lower stresses.[19] With reference to bending loads, both the cross-sectional area and bone tissue's distribution around a neutral axis are important geometric features. The area moment of inertia is the index that takes into account these two factors in bending. If the bone tissue is distributed further away from the neutral axis (the axis where the stresses and strains are zero) there is a larger area of inertia which means that it is more efficient in resisting bending (Fig. 1.3).

A bone's length also influences the bone's strength in bending. The longer the bone, the greater the magnitude of the bending moment caused by application of a force. For this reason, the lower extremity's long bones are subjected to high bending moments and therefore to high tensile and compressive stresses.[12]

Experiments in which standard-size bone specimens were used have shown that bones

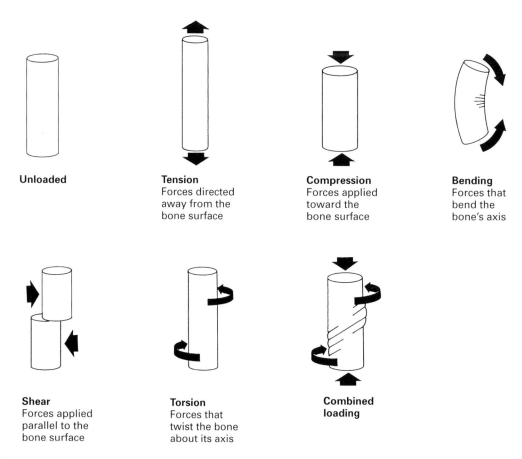

Fig. 1.1
Loading modes. (Adapted and reproduced, with permission, from Nordin M, Frankel VH. *Basic Biomechanics of the Musculoskeletal System*. Philadelphia: Lea & Febiger, 1989: 10.)

that have higher density are stronger.[20] Carter and Hayes[21] found that skeletal tissue's compressive strength is approximately proportional to the square of the apparent density. Their finding suggests that small reductions in bone density may be associated with large reductions in bone strength. Clinically, low bone density, which is measured using methods such as photon and X-ray absorptiometry and computed tomography, is associated with greater risk of osteoporotic fracture.[22]

When bone is loaded *in vivo*, contraction of muscles attached to bone also influences the stress magnitude and distribution. Nordsletten and colleagues found that intact soft tissues as well as muscle contraction substantially increase the rat tibia's structural capacity and that this effect is similar in normal and osteopenic bone.[23,24] Using biomechanical modeling, Scott and Winter[25] calculated the bending force acting on the tibia at a point one-third from the distal end during running. They found that the total force is a summation of the ground-reaction forces and the muscular forces. The greater positive bending moment created by the GRF was opposed by a smaller negative backward

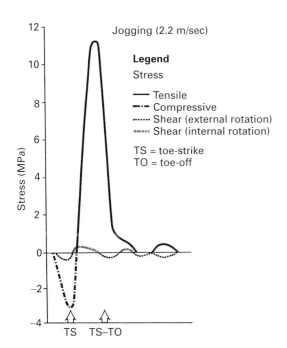

Fig. 1.2
Calculated stresses on the anteromedial cortex of a human tibia during jogging. (Adapted and reproduced, with permission, from Nordin M, Frankel VH. *Basic Biomechanics of the Musculoskeletal System.* Philadelphia: Lea & Febiger, 1989: 16.)

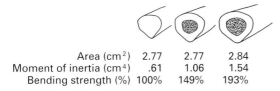

Area (cm²)	2.77	2.77	2.84
Moment of inertia (cm⁴)	.61	1.06	1.54
Bending strength (%)	100%	149%	193%

Fig. 1.3
Bone's moment-of-inertia properties. Although each of the three bones' cross-sectional areas are roughly equivalent, their bending strengths are very different because of differences in moments of inertia. This occurs as a result of the way the bone is distributed in relation to the central axis of bending or rotation. The solid bone on the left has the same amount of bone (area) as the one in the center, but the latter has higher moment of inertia because the bone is distributed further away from the central axis; its bending strength is therefore 50% greater. Similarly, the bone on the right has only slightly more bone than the one in the center, but its moment of inertia is again 50% higher; it is therefore 30% stronger under bending stress. (Adapted and reproduced, with permission, from Einhorn TA, Azria M, Goldstein SA. *Bone Fragility: The Biomechanics of Normal and Pathologic Bone, monograph.* Sandoz Pharma Ltd, 1992.)

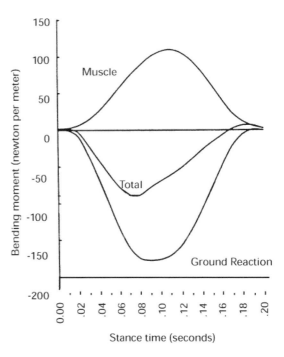

Fig. 1.4
Bending moment acting within the leg at a point one-third the distance from the distal tibial end. The total moment is the summation of the muscle and reaction bending moments. (Adapted and reproduced, with permission, from Scott SH, Winter DA. Internal forces at chronic running injury sites. *Medicine and Science in Sports and Exercise.* 1990; 22: 357–369.)

force created by the calf muscles as they acted to control the tibia's rotation and the foot's lowering to the ground (Fig. 1.4). Muscle activity therefore served to partially attenuate the large bending moment and to reduce the tensile and compressive stresses applied to the tibia. It therefore seems that muscle contraction can both decrease and increase the magnitude of stress applied to bone.

Normal response to load

Repetitive strains are essential for maintenance of normal bone mass. This fact is evident during situations of disuse, immobilization and weightlessness whereby dramatic bone loss occurs.[26,27] Physical activity can lead to increased bone mass because bone adapts to the additional loads placed on it.[28,29] However, bone can also lose strength as a result of repetitive loads imposed during normal daily activity. This loss of strength is attributed to formation and propagation of microscopic cracks within bone. If the load is continually applied, these 'microcracks' can spread and coalesce into 'macrocracks'. If repair does not occur, a stress fracture may eventually result.

Remodeling is a continuous, sequential process of breakdown and repair of microscopic cavities in bone. Remodeling occurs on both periosteal and endosteal surfaces within cortical bone and on the surface of trabeculae. The main functions of remodeling are:

1. to adapt bone to mechanical loading
2. to prevent accumulation of microfractures or fatigue damage
3. to maintain constant blood calcium levels.

Remodeling results in net bone resorption and is responsible for the bone losses that accompany aging.[30]

Both osteoclasts and osteoblasts are involved in remodeling and are organized into discrete packets named basic multicellular units (BMU). In human bone, the metabolic turnover rate is $0.05 \, mm^3$ of tissue every three to four months for each BMU. Following remodeling, bone requires three more months to mineralize sufficiently.[31]

Remodeling occurs in five stages:

1. quiescence
2. activation
3. resorption
4. reversal
5. formation.

A small area of bone surface is converted from rest to activity by an initiating stimulus, which may be hormonal, chemical, or physical. Osteoclast precursors are then recruited to the bone surface, where they fuse to form multinucleated osteoclasts.[32] These cells form a cavity by resorbing bone. A one- to two-week interval between termination of the resorptive processes and commencement of formation is known as the reversal phase. During this time, the bone site is weakened. Continued mechanical loading during the reversal phase could therefore result in microdamage accumulation and the beginning of clinical symptomatology.

Repair of the resorption cavity is performed by osteoblasts that accumulate within the cavity. Repair occurs in two stages: matrix synthesis and mineralization. First, a layer of bone matrix, known as an osteoid seam, is deposited. It mainly consists of Type I collagen and forms a three-dimensional scaffolding with which other bone-specific proteins may interact. After five to ten days of maturation, the new matrix begins to mineralize with crystals of hydroxyapatite that are deposited within and between the collagen fibrils. For this to occur, there must be an adequate supply of calcium and phosphate.[33]

Microdamage

Microdamage in bone tissue was first reported in 1951 by Rutishauser and Majno,[34] and later, in 1960, by Frost[35] when he observed cracks in nondecalcified sections of human rib bone. Since then, microscopy[36–38] and indirect techniques such as acoustic-emission[39,40] have revealed existence of bone microdamage following repetitive loading *in vivo*. Although hyperphysiological strain was used in many studies, microdamage has also been observed in bone subjected to physiological strain.[38,41] This suggests that microdamage may be a normal phenomenon in humans.

In vivo animal studies have provided substantial evidence of bone microdamage following repetitive loading.[42–46] For rabbits, two hours per day of forced jumping was sufficient to produce histologically identifiable cracks in the tibia after ten days.[44] With continued jumping, these cracks progressively accumulated and in some rabbits led to incomplete or complete tibial fractures. These findings were confirmed in another rabbit model because histologic microdamage was evident at sites that were subjected to repeated loading and that showed scintigraphic and radiologic evidence of tibial stress fracture.[45] Significant microdamage was produced in dog forelimbs subjected to three-point bending at 1500 or 2500 microstrain for 10,000 cycles.[43,46] However, lower strain magnitudes or fewer numbers of cycles did not produce significant bone microdamage.

These results suggest, first, that strains in the physiological range can initiate microdamage, thereby corroborating the findings of *in vitro* studies. Second, they suggest that a threshold level exists for accumulation of microdamage. Frost[47] also supports the concept of a microdamage threshold for bone. Based on fatigue, clinical and pathological studies, he suggests that this threshold is approximately 2000 microstrain, which represents the upper range of physiological values. He also hypothesizes that the relationship between strain and microdamage becomes exponential at deformations greater than 2000 microstrain.

Results of *in vivo* studies in which imaging techniques were used to detect microdamage in humans have differed. The differences most likely result from the fact that either the exercise period was insufficient for initiating microdamage[48] or the imaging may not have been sensitive enough.[49,50]

It is therefore reasonable to conclude that microdamage accumulates in human bone when repeated loading is undertaken. Frost[47] proposes classifying progression of bone microdamage into four stages. The molecular and ultrastructural stage is the earliest stage and may represent disruption of some intermolecular bonds in the mineralized matrix. Although this could correspond to a measurable loss of bone stiffness, this stage has not been directly visualized using microscopy. Increasing physical damage with wholesale disruption of molecular bonds may create prefailure planes in the previously impermeable mineralized matrix.

Although these planes do not appear as cracks under light microscopy, they enable large dye molecules such as basic fuschin to enter and can therefore be visualized using appropriate staining techniques. Accumulation and progression of prefailure planes may lead to frank physical cracks that are readily visible under the light microscope. The marked reduction in bone mechanical properties seen when repetitive loading is undertaken is attributed to these small cracks' formation. Increasing fatigue is associated with increased accumulation of cracks. When continued repetitive loading is undertaken, prefailure planes and cracks presumably accumulate and coalesce. At some stage they reach a critical size whereby so little bone remains to carry the imposed loads that a complete fracture finally occurs.

Response to excessive load

Because the threshold for bone microdamage seems to be within the upper range of normal activities, mechanisms must exist to prevent progression of microdamage. One mechanism is to limit crack propagation by virtue of the osteonal structure of Haversian bone. A second mechanism is the metabolic processes that exist in order to repair the damaged regions of bone.

The process of normal remodeling is thought to repair microdamage. Bone remodeling could repair microdamage in one of two ways: by directed repair, whereby the remodeling units are directed to the location of damage, or by simple random remodeling of the cortex at a rate designed to keep up with damage accumulation. Of the two ways, the theory of directed repair is favored by most researchers. However, for the directed repair to occur, there must be an initiating stimulus. Although the nature of this stimulus is not known, a cellular membrane response that results from disruption of osteocytes and the canalicular network has been suggested. Other researchers have claimed that the stimulus is an electrical response in the Haversian canal cells as a result of osteon debonding and cracking.

ACCELERATED REMODELING

As previously stated, normal remodeling, which is bone's response to cyclic loading is a sequential process of osteoclastic resorption and osteoblastic new-bone formation that occurs continuously on both periosteal and endosteal surfaces within cortical bone and on the surface of trabeculae.[2] Repetitive loads applied to bone that are below the single load failure threshold produce cumulative microdamage and initiate the process of accelerated remodeling. Microscopically, the first signs of accelerated remodeling are vascular congestion, thrombosis and osteoclastic resorption. When continued loading is undertaken, these findings progress to coalescence of resorbed cavities, and then to microfractures that extend to the cortex.

Histologic repair of microdamage was first documented in dogs. The researchers found increased osteoclastic and osteoblastic activity in fatigue-damaged regions[42] and significantly more microcracks in direct association with resorption spaces than had been expected by chance alone.[43] Although the studies show an association exists between microdamage and bone remodeling, they do not prove there is a cause-and-effect relationship.

That microdamage precedes or follows bone remodeling is unclear. Mori and Burr[46] demonstrated a significant increase in new remodeling events after bone microdamage was induced. Remodeling occurred preferentially in fatigue-damaged regions. However, there remained three times more resorption spaces than microcracks, and this suggests that factors other than microdamage also initiate remodeling. These factors include systemic and reproductive hormones, dietary factors, and bone strain that arises from mechanical loading.

Conversely, some human studies suggest that microdamage occurs at pre-existing sites of accelerated remodeling whereby osteoclastic resorption weakens an area of bone and subjects it to higher strains, before new bone is added by osteoblasts.[51–54] In a temporal series of stress-fracture biopsies mainly from the upper tibial cortex in humans, initial histology revealed accelerated cortical resorption.[53,55] Although no microfracture was seen at this stage, a thin crack was evident in many of the specimens a week later, followed by osteoblastic activity and new-bone formation. However, these studies do not reveal the exact timing of changes in response to loading. It is possible that microdamage was present before osteoclastic resorption but was histologically undetectable.

In the study by Li *et al.*,[44] an exercising rabbit model was used in order to assess sequential pathologic changes in the tibia's internal structure that were caused by controlled excessive physical activity during a ten-week period. Rabbits were induced to jump and run 360 times per day during a two-hour session whereby the researchers were able to control the loading regimen's intensity, duration and interval. During the ten-week period, animals were sacrificed at intervals, and histologic features were recorded. As early as day two, vascular and circulatory disturbances, including engorgement, vasodilation and hyaline thrombosis were evident. Within the first week, collagen fibers were forming in the periosteum, there was osteocyte shrinkage and necrosis, and osteoclast and resorption cavities were generated in the tibial cortex and interstitial lamellae.

It was not until the second week that small cracks appeared at the cement line of the Haversian system. At this stage, there was obvious osteoclastic resorption and a large number of cavity formations, together with increasing subperiosteal osteoblast activity and periosteal proliferation. By the third week, incomplete fracture of the tibial cortex was found in some specimens and seemed to be the result of convergence of several neighboring cracks in the Haversian system. New-bone formation reached a maximum after twenty-one days. Remodeling continued in both the newly formed bone and the original bone of the tibial cortex, and there was an increase in capillaries and development of structures that resembled the Haversian canal.

Over the remaining six weeks, the resorption cavities were gradually filled in with new bone by osteoblasts and then converted to Haversian bone. Periosteal new bone and the original bone fused during the remodeling process and thereby thickened the tibial cortex. One specimen developed a cortical fracture. Although most tibiae therefore successfully adapt to changes in bone strain as a result of repetitive loading, through internal remodeling, fractures may appear if excessive stress continues in a tibia weakened by osteoclastic resorption.

Clinical presentation of stress fractures follows a continuum that closely reflects the accelerated remodeling occurring in the bone. Accelerated remodeling does not at first produce symptoms, and plain radiographs will be normal, although magnetic resonance imaging (MRI) may show marrow edema, and nuclear bone scan will show focal uptake of technetium. As accelerated remodeling progresses, mild pain will occur some time after the onset of exercise and will, with further progression, occur earlier in the exercise bout. If loading does not cease, pain intensity will increase and will be present even after the exercise bout and during normal activities involved in daily living. At this point, a technetium bone scan will be positive in all three phases and MRI will show marrow edema, but plain radiographs, which specifically detect new bone formation or complete fractures, will remain negative. By the time plain radiographs are positive, a full-blown stress fracture is present. It is important to realize that this process is on a continuum both physiologically and clinically and that early intervention is associated with more-rapid healing.

Clinical correlations

From a clinical point of view, five factors are usually assessed in relation to pathogenesis of a stress fracture. Within the clinical arena, these factors have moved from tenets to dogma over the past two decades. Although evidence substantiating the causal relationship between these factors and stress fractures is lacking (this will be discussed in Chapter 3), clinical experience indicates that the factors are of value in treatment of stress fractures.

TRAINING ERRORS

Training errors – increases in physical activity (bone loading) at a rate that exceeds the rate of remodeling in bone – are the most important factor. The expression 'Too much too soon' includes the total load and the intensity or pace. A sudden increase in either, or resumption of a high level of activity after a prolonged layoff period, is often associated with development of a stress fracture. Training errors are most important in the case of and are often associated with onset of stress fractures in nonelite, recreational athletes.

MUSCLE FATIGUE

Muscle fatigue may also be an important factor in stress-fracture pathogenesis. Attenuation of ground-reaction forces mainly through eccentric contraction of muscle minimizes the load transmitted to bone. If muscle fatigue occurs during an exercise bout, bone will experience greater load. Clinical measurement of muscular strength does not typically measure muscle's fatiguability; the latter is metabolic ability to sustain effective muscular contractions by continuously producing adenosine triphosphate through oxidative phosphorylation at the rate required to sustain a given workload. Muscular resistance to fatigue occurs through sport-specific training and muscular adaptations that provide enhanced oxidative capacity. Although these adaptations require a minimum of eight weeks' training, improvements in fatiguability resistance in fact increase for many months when training is undertaken.

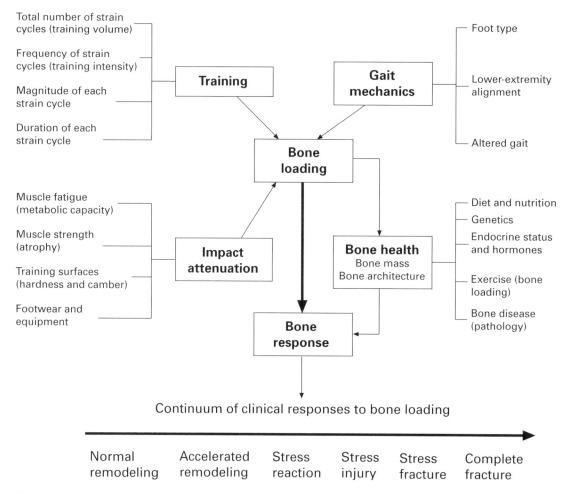

Fig. 1.5

Training influences bone loading and is itself affected by four factors. The volume of training is a function of the total number of strain cycles received by the bone, and the intensity of training (load per unit time: pace, or speed) is a function of the frequency of strain cycles applied to the bone. The magnitude of each strain and duration of each strain cycle are a function of body weight, muscular shock-absorption capability, and lower-extremity biomechanic alignment. Impact attenuation is both intrinsic (muscular factors) and extrinsic (equipment and training surfaces). Although eccentric muscular strength is important, even more important is the muscle's ability to resist fatigue: to continue to contract effectively for a sustained period of time. This important factor is a function of metabolic adaptations that occur when training is undertaken. Although foot type and lower-extremity biomechanical alignment may affect gait mechanics, altered gait may also occur from fatigue, disease, and injury. Finally, bone health is a major factor that determines bone's response to loading and is affected by diet and nutrition, genetics, endocrine and hormonal status, amount of regular exercise, and presence of bone disease.

LOWER-EXTREMITY ALIGNMENT

Lower-extremity alignment is a third factor that likely predisposes a person to development of stress fractures. Highly arched, pes-cavus feet absorb less shock whereas pes-planus feet transmit more force to the tibia. Genu varum and valgum, excessive Q angles, leg-length discrepancies, and femoral-neck anteversion are all associated with variations in gait that can influence force distribution to bone in the lower extremity.

TERRAIN

Terrain, the fourth factor, influences force delivered to bone in two ways. Hard surfaces require greater shock absorption by lower-leg muscles, and cambered or uneven surfaces require compensatory muscular contractions that alter the balance of loading between the two lower extremities.

EQUIPMENT

Equipment, especially footwear, can influence the load delivered to bone both in relation to a shock-absorption standpoint and with reference to whether or not the design accommodates foot type and lower-extremity alignment.

Clinical response to bone loading can be correlated with the mechanical and cellular responses (Fig. 1.5). Mechanical factors that contribute to stress fracture include the absolute number of strain cycles (volume of training, and total accumulative load), the frequency of the strain cycles (load per unit time: the intensity, and pace), the magnitude of strain in each load cycle (factors that affect shock absorption and shock attenuation, including muscular strength and endurance, footwear, and lower-extremity alignment), and duration of each strain cycle (terrain, lower-extremity alignment, and footwear).

Clinical response of bone to load can be seen along a continuum, from accelerated remodeling to a complete stress fracture. Symptomatology, physical-examination findings, and the results of radiographic-imaging studies will be a function of the extent of the injury's progression along the continuum.

References

1 Cowin SC, Moss-Salentijn L, Moss ML. Candidates for the mechanosensory system in bone. *Journal of Biomechanical Engineering* 1991; 113: 191–197.

2 Buckwalter JA, Glimcher MJ, Cooper RR, Recker R. Bone biology. *Journal of Bone and Joint Surgery* 1995; 77-A: 1256–1275.

3 Boivin G, Anthoine-Terrier C, Obrant KJ. Transmission electron microscopy of bone tissue. *Acta Orthopaedica Scandinavica* 1990; 61: 170–180.

4 Peck WA, Woods WL. The cells of bone. In: Riggs BL, Melton LJ, eds. *Osteoporosis: Etiology, Diagnosis, and Management.* New York: Raven Press, 1988: 1–44.

5 Cavanagh PR, LaFortune MA. Ground reaction forces in distance running. *Journal of Biomechanics* 1980; 13: 397–406.

6 McNitt-Gray J. Kinematics and impulse characteristics of drop landings from three heights. *International Journal of Sports Biomechanics* 1991; 7: 201–223.

7 Light LH, McLellan GE, Klenerman L. Skeletal transients on heel strike in normal walking with different footwear. *Journal of Biomechanics* 1980; 13: 477–480.

8 Wosk J, Voloshin A. Wave attenuation in skeletons of young healthy persons. *Journal of Biomechanics* 1981; 14: 261–267.

9 Hamill J, Bates BT, Knutzen KM, Sawhill JA. Variations in ground reaction force parameters at different running speeds. *Human Movement Science* 1983; 2: 47–56.

10 Nigg BM, Segesser B. The influence of playing surfaces on the load on the locomotor system and on football and tennis injuries. *Sports Medicine* 1988; 5: 375–385.

11 Dufek JS, Bates BT. Dynamic performance assessment of selected sport shoes on impact forces. *Medicine and Science in Sports and Exercise* 1991; 23: 1062–1067.

12 Nordin M, Frankel VH. *Basic Biomechanics of the Musculoskeletal System*, 2nd edn. Philadelphia: Lea & Febiger, 1989.

13 Einhorn TA. Biomechanics of bone. In: Bilezikian JP, Raisz LG, Rodan GA, eds. *Principles of Bone Biology*. San Diego: Academic Press, 1996.

14 Lanyon LE, Hampson WGJ, Goodship AE, Shah JS. Bone deformation recorded *in vivo* from strain gauges attached to the human tibial shaft. *Acta Orthopaedica Scandinavica* 1975; 46: 256–268.

15 Burr DB, Milgrom C, Fyhrie D *et al. In vivo* measurement of human tibial strains during vigorous activity. *Bone* 1996; 18: 405–410.

16 Ekenman I, Halvorsen K, Westblad P, Fellandertsai L, Rolf C. Local bone deformation at two predominant sites for stress fractures of the tibia: an *in vivo* study. *Foot and Ankle International* 1998; 19: 479–484.

17 Milgrom C, Burr D, Fyhrie D *et al.* A comparison of the effect of shoes in human tibial axial strains recorded during dynamic loading. *Foot and Ankle International* 1998; 19: 85–90.

18 Carter DR. Anisotropic analysis of strain rosette information from cortical bone. *Journal of Biomechanics* 1978; 11: 199–202.

19 Hayes WC, Gerhart TN. Biomechanics of bone: applications for assessment of bone strength. *Bone and Mineral Research* 1985; 3: 259–294.

20 Alho A, Husby T, Hoiseth A. Bone mineral content and mechanical strength. An *ex vivo* study on human femora at autopsy. *Clinical Orthopaedics and Related Research* 1986; 227: 292–297.

21 Carter DR, Hayes WC. The compressive behavior of bone as a two-phase porous structure. *Journal of Bone and Joint Surgery* 1977; 59-A: 954–962.

22 Cummings SR, Black DM, Nevitt MC *et al.* Bone density at various sites for prediction of hip fractures. *Lancet* 1993; 341: 72–75.

23 Nordsletten L, Ekeland A. Muscle contraction increases the structural capacity of the lower leg: an *in vivo* study in the rat. *Journal of Orthopaedic Research* 1993; 11: 299–304.

24 Nordsletten L, Kaastad TS, Obrant KJ *et al.* Muscle contraction increases the *in vivo* structural strength to the same degree in osteopenic and normal rat tibiae. *Journal of Bone and Mineral Research* 1994; 9: 679–685.

25 Scott SH, Winter DA. Internal forces at chronic running injury sites. *Medicine and Science in Sports and Exercise* 1990; 22: 357–369.

26 Whedon GD. Disuse osteoporosis: physiological aspects. *Calcified Tissue International* 1984; 36: S146–S150.

27 Hamdy RC, Krishnaswamy G, Cancellaro V, Whalen K, Harvill L. Changes in bone mineral content and density after stroke. *American Journal of Physical Medicine and Rehabilitation* 1993; 72: 188–191.

28 Morris FL, Naughton GA, Gibbs JL, Carlson JS, Wark JD. Prospective ten-month exercise intervention in premenarcheal girls: positive effects on bone and lean mass. *Journal of Bone and Mineral Research* 1997; 12: 1453–1462.

29 Bass S, Pearce G, Bradney M *et al.* Exercise before puberty may confer residual benefits in bone density in adulthood: studies in active prepubertal and retired female gymnasts. *Journal of Bone and Mineral Research* 1998; 13: 500–507.

30 Marcus R. Skeletal aging: understanding the functional and structural basis of osteoporosis. *Trends in Endocrinology and Metabolism* 1991; 2: 53–58.

31 Frost HM. Some ABC's of skeletal pathophysiology. 6. The growth/modeling/remodeling distinction. *Calcified Tissue International* 1991; 49: 301–302.

32 Parfitt AM. The three organizational levels of bone remodelling: implications for the interpretation of biochemical markers and the mechanisms of bone loss. In: Christiansen C, Overgaard K, eds. *Osteoporosis* 1990. Copenhagen: Osteopress, 1990: 429–434.

33 Parfitt AM. Bone remodeling: relationship to the amount and structure of bone, and the pathogenesis and prevention of fractures. In: Riggs BL, Melton LJ, eds. *Osteoporosis: Etiology, Diagnosis, and Management.* New York: Raven Press, 1988.

34 Rutishauser E, Majno G. Physiopathology of bone tissue: the osteocytes and fundamental substance. *Bulletin of the Hospital for Joint Diseases* 1951; 12: 468–490.

35 Frost HL. Presence of microscopic cracks *in vivo* in bone. *Henry Ford Hospital Medical Bulletin* 1960; 8: 25–35.

36 Carter DR, Hayes WC. Compact bone fatigue damage-1. Residual strength and stiffness. *Journal of Biomechanics* 1977; 10: 325–337.

37 Forwood MR, Parker AW. Microdamage in response to repetitive torsional loading in the rat tibia. *Calcified Tissue International* 1989; 45: 47–53.

38 Schaffler MB, Radin EL, Burr DB. Long-term fatigue behavior of compact bone at low strain magnitude and rate. *Bone* 1990; 11: 321–326.

39 Netz P, Eriksson K, Stromberg L. Material reaction of diaphyseal bone under torsion. *Acta Orthopaedica Scandinavica* 1980; 51: 223–229.

40 Jonsson U, Eriksson K. Microcracking in dog bone under load. *Acta Orthopaedica Scandanavica* 1984; 55: 441–445.

41 Schaffler MB, Radin EL, Burr DB. Mechanical and morphological effects of strain rate on fatigue of compact bone. *Bone* 1989; 10: 207–214.

42 Chamay A, Tschantz P. Mechanical influences in bone remodeling: experimental research on Wolff's law. *Journal of Biomechanics* 1972; 5: 173–180.

43 Burr DB, Martin RB, Schaffler MB, Radin EL. Bone remodeling in response to *in vivo* fatigue microdamage. *Journal of Biomechanics* 1985; 18: 189–200.

44 Li G, Zhang S, Chen G, Chen H, Wang A. Radiographic and histologic analyses of stress fracture in rabbit tibias. *American Journal of Sports Medicine* 1985; 13: 285–294.

45 Burr DB, Milgrom C, Boyd RD *et al.* Experimental stress fractures of the tibia. *Journal of Bone and Joint Surgery* 1990; 72: 370–375.

46 Mori S, Burr DB. Increased intracortical remodeling following fatigue damage. *Bone* 1993; 14: 103–109.

47 Frost HM. Transient-steady state phenomena in microdamage physiology: a proposed algorithm for lamellar bone. *Calcified Tissue International* 1989; 44; 367–381.

48 Forwood MR, Parker AW. Repetitive loading, *in vivo*, of the tibia and femora of rats: effects of a single bout of treadmill running. *Calcified Tissue International* 1992; 50: 193–196.

49 Rubin CT, Pratt GW, Porter AL, Lanyon LE, Poss R. The use of ultrasound *in vivo* to determine acute change in the mechanical properties of bone following intense physical activity. *Journal of Biomechanics* 1987; 20: 723–727.

50 Bennell KL, Hart P, Nattrass C, Wark JD. Acute and subacute changes in the ultrasound measurements of the calcaneus following intense exercise. *Calcified Tissue International* 1998; 63: 505–509.

51 Straus FH. Marching fractures of metatarsal bones with a report of the pathology. *Surgery, Gynecology and Obstetrics* 1932; 54: 581–584.

52 Burrows HJ. Fatigue infraction of the middle of the tibia in ballet dancers. *Journal of Bone and Joint Surgery* 1956; 38B: 83–94.

53 Johnson LC, Stradford HT, Geis RW, Dineen JR, Kerley E. Histogenesis of stress fractures. *Journal of Bone and Joint Surgery* 1963; 45A: 1542.

54 Michael RH, Holder LE. The soleus syndrome: a cause of medial tibial stress (shin splints). *American Journal of Sports Medicine* 1985; 13: 87–94.

55 Jones H, Harris JM, Vinh TN, Rubin C. Exercise-induced stress fractures and stress reactions of bone: epidemiology, etiology, and classification. *Exercise and Sports Sciences Review* 1989; 17: 379–422.

Chapter 2

The epidemiology of stress fractures

*T*he literature is full of case reports about stress fractures that have occurred in association with virtually every type of sport and physical activity. Even if rigorously conducted clinical trials or cohort studies have not been undertaken, a sagacious person would conclude that stress fractures are by far most common in the lower extremity and in weightbearing activities, particularly activities that involve running or jumping. Although this is true, the fractures also occur in the upper extremity and in non-weightbearing activities such as swimming and throwing. Information about the frequency, incidence, and prevalence of stress fractures, in various sports that have various training regimens, and in various clinical situations, in both men and women, is essential for prediction and prevention of injury.

At the time of this writing, however, as might be expected, the literature about stress fractures in athletes is heterogeneous with reference to study design, subject pools, treatments, and outcome-measurement tools. For this reason, it is difficult to make valid comparisons for the purpose of risk-factor identification, training recommendations, and clinical interventions. However, enough descriptive data are available to enable conclusions to be drawn in some areas and inferences to be made in others. In this chapter, the descriptive epidemiology of stress fractures is reviewed.

Methodology issues

In order to review the epidemiological data about stress fractures, including injury rates, injury characteristics, and injury morbidity, we must begin by briefly discussing specific issues related to published studies' methodology.

In the basic sciences, research methods and techniques are used that serve to carefully isolate the factors under study (independent variables) and the outcomes being measured (dependent variables). This type of research serves to unravel individual questions within the much larger sphere of the overall problem. By comparison, clinical research is often viewed as being more relevant, more immediate, and more

generalizable to the clinical condition under study. However, clinical research lacks precision; confounding or extraneous variables are many, and error terms are large. Results often remain open to speculation if underlying mechanisms remain elusive or if threats to validity remain unanswered. In a way, basic science excels in its sensitivity whereas clinical science excels in its specificity. Although arguments favoring both approaches are common, reality would indicate that a combination of both would yield the most accurate research information.

As is the case with any clinical study, ability to make valid conclusions about stress-fracture morbidity and treatment depends on the study design used, the presence of potential confounding elements, and additional factors that may influence bias or chance. In clinical studies of stress fracture, the single-most important goal is to establish causal relationships; in other words, the validity of the conclusions made from clinical studies is determined by the extent to which the relationships between a given set of variables is able to show cause and effect. Causality is exceedingly important in establishing whether a given association is valid, and, by extension, whether an intervention might be effective.

STUDY DESIGN

Generally, the following six types of research design have been used in study of stress fractures.

CLINICAL TRIALS

These types of study are best used for evaluating treatment strategies once stress fractures have occurred. They are the clinical equivalent of an experiment. The researcher takes an active role by applying some intervention to the subjects. In a true clinical trial, the intervention or treatment is applied to randomly selected cases, and the nonselected cases form the control group. Random selection helps distribute any extraneous variables equally between the treatment and control group, and any potential confounding is thereby eliminated.

The clinical trial is best suited to measuring a treatment's efficacy or effectiveness in changing stress fractures' natural history. A clinical trial may also be conducted in order to assess injury-prevention strategies. However, if a study's goal is to understand stress fractures' cause (usually by gaining an understanding of the risk factors for injury), an observational design is best used. The remaining five types of study design are considered to be 'observational' in that they involve making observations about injuries and related factors without taking an

active role in the process. They are ideal for understanding stress fractures' natural history and can be used to uncover injury cause.

PROSPECTIVE COHORT STUDIES

In these types of study, participants are assembled at the beginning of the study according to their exposure to some (risk) factor. All the participants are followed over a predetermined length of time, during which injury occurrence is monitored and recorded by way of some form of surveillance. This type of study is a 'strong' design because it enables accurate comparisons to be made between injured and noninjured groups. From these comparisons, a true assessment of incidence and risk can be made, and causal inferences drawn.

Although a number of prospective cohort studies in athletes have been undertaken that evaluated incidence rates for all injuries or for broad categories of injuries (for example sprains and strains), only a few specifically evaluated stress fractures. By contrast, the military literature contains numerous prospective cohort studies that investigated stress-fracture incidence rates.

Reasons abound as to why few studies of this type exist in the civilian stress-fracture literature. In order to have enough statistical power, particularly for detection of small differences, sample sizes have to be quite large, and this need may be difficult to meet at a single center if stress fractures are uncommon. Rigorous inclusion criteria and dropout rates over the course of the study also limit the number of available, suitable subjects.

A variation on the prospective cohort design is the *historical cohort design*. Although it is a cohort study because its 'starting point' is classification of subjects into exposed and nonexposed groups, this initial exposure classification is based on data previously collected (for example from historical records). These groups have already been exposed to risk of injury before the time the data are collected, and stress fractures have already been sustained by some of the subjects some time in the past.

Both prospective and historical cohort studies enable the relative risk of injury to be calculated in the participants exposed versus the ones not exposed to some risk factor.

CASE–CONTROL STUDIES

These types of study differ from the cohort types in that participants are assembled according to whether or not they have sustained a stress fracture, whereby the injured subjects form the cases and the noninjured subjects form the controls. The prior exposure to some risk factor is then ascertained in each group. Stress-fracture rates can be calculated, because the design involves both numerator (number of injuries) and denominator (exposure) data.

However, data about stress-fracture rates from these types of study may be biased as a result of selection factors that affect subject enrolment and as a result of inaccurate recall of prior exposure. Because many confounders, such as gender, age, menstrual status, and activity can affect the studies, cases and controls are often matched on one or more of these variables. When extraneous variables are accounted for, the study can more accurately determine the impact of the risk factors under investigation. In contrast to cohort studies, the case–control design enables risk to be calculated as an odds of exposure (to some risk factor) in the injured (case) compared with the noninjured (control) subjects.

CASE SERIES

These are single-study groups that comprise individuals who have a stress fracture and who usually present to a clinic or another treatment facility. The main value of case series is that they enable stress fractures' relative frequency to be compared with other injuries in the same population of patients. They can also be used for describing various characteristics of both the stress fracture and the injured athlete, giving a general indication of morbidity, and generating hypotheses about etiology and treatment.

Case series is the type of study design most commonly found in the stress-fracture literature, because of the existence of convenient access to a clinical database for the study population. However, because case-series designs do not provide information about the population from which the injuries arose (absence of denominator data), they cannot be used for calculating the true incidence of stress fracture, drawing inferences about risk of injury, postulating mechanisms related to stress fractures' etiology or pathophysiology, or assessing treatment regimens.

Because the composition of most case series strongly reflects various selection and referral mechanisms, this results in a nonrepresentative sample population,[1] and introduction of sample bias. Although the single-case report can often be clinically instructive and detailed with reference to an unusual stress fracture or clinical presentation, it cannot be used for forming any conclusions about incidence, treatment, or morbidity. Most of the nonmilitary stress-fracture literature comprises case series and case reports that provide detailed clinical commentary and at least preliminary insights into the morbidity and effectiveness of various clinical-treatment protocols. However, many unanswered questions remain about stress fractures' etiology and pathogenesis that require investigation using more-rigorous study designs.

CROSS-SECTIONAL STUDIES, OR SURVEYS

These studies also have elements in common with case-control and cohort studies in that they can document presence of risk factors ('exposure') and of stress fractures ('outcome'). However, because presence of the risk factor and of the stress fracture are measured at the same point in time, these studies cannot show whether the risk factor preceded the stress fracture's development. Because a temporal relationship cannot be established, it is not possible to know whether a (risk) factor caused or contributed to a stress fracture's development or whether it was merely the result of the stress fracture. Therefore, although these studies are informative, they cannot establish cause-and-effect relationships.

'MIXED' STUDY DESIGNS

In these studies, elements from the case series and cohort designs are combined. An example is a study that documents injury occurrence at a road race whereby the runners who register for the event define the cohort. Because detailed information would not be available for noninjured runners, this approach does not represent a true cohort design. However, because the number of runners exposed to the possibility of injury can be determined, the design does provide data about injury rates: a measure that cannot be estimated in a case-series design.

These studies' findings are generalizable only to people who participate in road-race events. Also, they typically rely on self-reporting; therefore, injured athletes who commonly do not seek attention at events will not be included in the study, and this results in what can be a considerable underestimation of the injury's frequency.

STUDY INTERPRETATION

Apart from the study design, a number of factors can influence interpretation of the results and of the conclusions' validity. The most common factors are confounding, sampling methods, sample size, expression of incidence rates, length of stress-fracture observation period, dropouts, and the clinical definition of stress fracture.

In consolidating the findings of any group of studies, the key factor is interpretation of any conclusions' validity. Caution is required, because the (confounding) factors that affect ability to draw conclusions tend to be specific to the problem under study. Stress-fracture investigations are no exception, and have been confounded by a number of factors.

Confounding has been defined as a mixing of the effect of the exposure under study on the disease under study with that of a third factor.[2] The difficulty involved in confounding is therefore that an observed association between any two variables of interest could either totally or in part be the result of the effects of a third variable. Two conditions must be satisfied for confounding to exist. First, the third factor must be associated with the exposure, and second, independent of that exposure, be a risk factor for the disease.[2] The net effect of confounding is that the observed association between some factor and disease can be attributed to the confounder's effect. It can lead to an over- or underestimation of a factor's effect, or even change the direction of the observed association.

Confounding rarely adds to our understanding of injury cause, because it is a property of a specific study rather than a function of the actual injury process. Refer to Meeuwisse[3] for a more detailed description of this important concept.

A second major cause of bias is the selection factors that affect subject enrolment. For example, if nonrandom sampling is used for recruiting subjects, the people who choose to enrol may be different in several important ways from the people who do not enrol. For example, body-composition factors associated with success in competition may also be factors whereby the athlete is placed at risk for stress-fracture development. A nonrandom sample may have systematic characteristics apart from the stress fracture that are different from those of a random sample and that may influence stress-fracture risk independently. Athlete stress-fracture studies often comprise small sample sizes, and this limits generalizability to the larger, active population. By comparison, military populations lend themselves well to data collection and enable much larger samples to be studied. However, given the differences in training, footwear and initial fitness levels, the results from military studies are usually not generalizable to civilian athlete populations.

The two main measures of injury frequency are prevalence and incidence. Prevalence quantifies the proportion of individuals in a population who have a stress fracture at a specific point in time. Incidence quantifies the rate of new stress fractures that develop in a population of individuals who are at risk during a specific time or exposure interval.[2] Incidence is the more widely used measure in the stress-fracture literature.

The way in which incidence is expressed in the stress-fracture literature differs, depending on the way in which numerator and denominator data are calculated. In some studies, 'participant rates' are reported whereby the total number of athletes (or recruits) who have a stress fracture is divided by the total number of participants. A difficulty involved in this approach is that athletes may develop more than one stress fracture either concurrently or at another time. An alternative is to calculate 'case rates' whereby the numerator consists of the total number of stress fractures that occur during the study period. In practise, participant and case rates are often presented as a percentage, that is, the number of athletes who have a stress fracture or the number of stress fractures per 100 athletes. However, in some studies it is difficult to tell whether case or participant rates have been presented. The results are often further broken down and calculated according to participant characteristics such as age, gender, and competitive level. This method is useful because these characteristics may influence stress-fracture rates, but it is often not possible to be used because of small sample sizes.

The length of stress-fracture observation periods differs between studies. In the military, most researchers calculate stress-fracture rates during eight- to twelve-week training periods.

This may be an appropriate time interval for some types of fracture but not for others. For studies in athletes, varying time periods are used. The most common method has been to assess whether or not participants have ever sustained one or more stress fractures at any time in the past. Strictly speaking, this provides neither an incidence rate nor a prevalence rate, because the observation period is not taken into consideration and is inconsistent between individuals.

Expression of stress-fracture rates as participant or case rates may not enable a meaningful comparison to be made of the results of various studies either within the same sport or between sports. Participants' varying exposure to stress-fracture risk can lead to inaccurate denominator data. For example, a player who is sidelined is not at the same risk of sustaining a stress fracture as one who plays the entire season. Likewise, someone who runs three miles per week for six months is not at the same risk as someone who runs fifty miles per week over the same period. In the more recent injury literature, methods have been introduced for quantifying exposure, and examples include expressing rates in terms of practise matches, long jumps, or hours of running.[4] To date, only two civilian stress-fracture studies have expressed incidence rates in terms of exposure.[5,6]

In longer-term studies or less controlled environments, subjects may drop out of a study. This is of concern particularly in cohort studies or clinical trials. If the people who drop out have characteristics (for example age, gender, and severity or site of the stress fracture) different from the ones of the people who stay in the study, significant biases may be introduced.

Another potential problem is the fact that the clinical definition of stress fracture varies from center to center, and from study to study. This naturally has a great influence on reporting of stress-fracture incidence and prevalence rates as well as of stress-fracture site distributions, and this presents a substantial limitation to comparison of studies. For example, some studies rely on radiographic confirmation whereas others use bone scan or other imaging data, and others again place the greatest emphasis on clinical findings. Given plain radiographs' relative insensitivity for stress-fracture diagnosis, in studies that use them as a diagnostic criterion the true stress-fracture incidence will be seriously underestimated. Conversely, bone scans have great sensitivity but reduced specificity, and if they are relied on as a diagnostic criterion the true stress-fracture incidence will be overestimated.

Despite the abovementioned considerations, it is important it be pointed out that the limitations inherent in stress-fracture studies are similar to those found in virtually all clinical research. The field of sports medicine is relatively new, and over the past decade we have witnessed a considerable improvement in the quality of research and published studies. Enough published data are now available to enable useful insights to be gained into various aspects related to stress-fracture morbidity.

Stress-fracture rates in specific sports

The current literature with reference to the rate of stress-fracture occurrence in the nonmilitary population is summarized in Table 2.1.[5–21] Specific details and conclusions made from these studies are discussed as follows in a sequence the same as that for the studies set out in Table 2.1.

In the studies to date, variation in reported rates probably reflects differences in cohort demographics, including the subjects' sex and age, and in methodology, including the study design, the definition of stress fracture used and the timeframe of observation. Most of the literature is about elite-, competitive- or professional-level athletes and contains little information about stress-fracture rates during recreational or occupational physical activity. One recent study did compare the lifetime frequency of medically diagnosed stress fractures in 2298 collegiate athletes and 683 collegiate nonathletes using a self-administered questionnaire.[21] As expected, athletes had a significantly greater frequency, and figures for women were given as 25% in athletes and 15% in nonathletes. Although this stress-fracture rate may seem to be high for nonathletes, the individuals' exercise history was not evaluated, and the questionnaire's response rate was only 43%, which was much lower than the 97% response rate for athletes. The noninjured, non-athletes may therefore not have been as likely as their injured counterparts to return the questionnaires.

COLLEGIATE SPORT

A retrospective review of the medical records of 207 female collegiate athletes showed a 6.5% incidence of stress fractures confirmed in one year by way of X-ray.[7] In fact the figure may be an underestimate of the problem, because X-rays are not always positive even though a fracture may exist. Although this study did not break down the results according to individual sports, two other studies do enable stress-fracture rates in various collegiate athletes to be compared (Table 2.2).

Goldberg and Pecora[17] reviewed the medical records of collegiate athletes over a three-year period. Approximate participant numbers were available in order to enable incidence of stress-fracture case rates in each sport to be estimated, but data from men and women were combined. The highest annual incidence occurred in softball (6.3%), followed by track (3.7%), basketball (2.9%), tennis (2.8%), gymnastics (2.8%), lacrosse (2.7%), baseball (2.7%), and crew (2.2%). These figures should be viewed as being only approximate, because participant numbers were small in some sports, and this may reduce the findings' validity.

Similar results were reported by Johnson et al.,[18] who conducted a two-year prospective

Table 2.1 Rates of stress-fracture incidence in athletes, expressed as a participant percentage rate unless otherwise indicated

Reference	Study design	Population	Subjects	Data collection method	Questionnaire response rate	Observation period	Diagnosis of stress fracture	Stress-fracture rate
Collegiate sport								
Lloyd et al. 1986[7]	XS	Collegiate athletes	207 – F	Review of medical records	NA	1 year	X-ray	6.5%†
Goldberg and Pecora 1994[17]	CS	Collegiate athletes	≈ 1200 – F ≈ 1800 – M	Review of medical records	NA	3 years	X-ray or BS	2.7% – F†# 1.4% – M†#
Johnson et al. 1994[18]	PC	Collegiate athletes	321 – F 593 – M	Monitoring	NA	2 years	X-ray or BS	6.9% – F†# 2.0% – M†#
Nattiv et al. 1997[21]	XS	Collegiate athletes	738 – F 1502 – M	Self-administered questionnaire	97%	Hx	NS	25.0% – F NS – M
Running								
Barrow and Saha 1988[9]	XS	Collegiate distance runners	240 – F	Self-administered questionnaire	24%	Hx	X-ray or BS	37.0%
Collins et al. 1989[10]	XS	Finishers in Seafair Triathlon	198 – M 59 – F	Self-administered questionnaire	45%	1 year	NS	3.5% – M 3.4% – F
Brunet et al. 1990[12]	XS	Recreational and competitive runners	375 – F 1130 – M	Self-administered questionnaire	NS	Hx	NS	13.2% – F 8.3% – M
Goldberg and Pecora 1994[17]	CS	Collegiate athletes	≈ 486 – F and M	Review of medical records	NA	3 years	X-ray or BS	3.7%†#
Johnson et al. 1994[18]	PC	Track athletes	45 – F 62 – M	Monitoring	NA	2 years	X-ray or BS	31.1%– F† 9.7% – M†#
Bennell et al. 1995[19]	XS	Track and field athletes	53 – F	Self-administered questionnaire	100%	Hx	X-ray, BS, or CT	51.5% 84.9%#
Bennell et al. 1996[5]	PC	Track and field athletes	46 – F 49 – M	Monitoring	NA	1 year	BS and CT	21.7% – F† 20.4% – M† 30.4% – F†# 24.5% – M†#
Ballet dancing								
Warren et al. 1986[8]	CC	Professional ballet dancers	40 – F	Self-administered questionnaire	100%	Hx	X-ray or BS	45.0% 67.5%#
Frusztajer et al. 1990[13]	CC	Ballet dancers	45 – F	Interview and questionnaire	100%	1 year	NS	22.0%†
Kadel et al. 1992[15]	XS	Professional ballet dancers	54 – F	Self-administered questionnaire	100%	Hx	X-ray or BS	31.5% 50.0%#

Table 2.1 continues.

Table 2.1 continued

Reference	Study design	Population	Subjects	Data collection method	Questionnaire response rate	Observation period	Diagnosis of stress fracture	Stress-fracture rate
Figure skating								
Pecina et al. 1990[14]	XS	Elite ice skaters	42 M and F	Self-administered questionnaire	100%	Hx	NS	21.0%
Gymnastics								
Dixon and Fricker 1993[16]	CS	Elite: holders of scholarship	74 – F 42 – M	Review of medical records	NA	10 years	X-ray or BS	27.0% – F# 14.3% – M#
Goldberg and Pecora 1994[17]	CS	Collegiate athletes	≈ 36 – M and F	Review of medical records	NA	3 years	X-ray or BS	2.8%†#
Crew								
Reid et al. 1989[11]	CS	Elite	40 – F	Review of medical records	NA	4 years	NS	7.5%#
Goldberg and Pecora 1994[17]	CS	Collegiate athletes	≈ 495 – M and F	Review of medical records	NA	3 years	X-ray or BS	2.2%†#
Johnson et al. 1994[18]	PC	Collegiate athletes	49 – F 42 – M	Monitoring	NA	2 years	X-ray or BS	8.2% – F† 2.4% – M†
Hickey et al. 1997[6]	CS	Elite: holders of scholarship	84 – F 88 – M	Review of medical records	NA	10 years	NS	17.9% – F 3.4% – M
Basketball								
Goldberg and Pecora 1994[17]	CS	Collegiate athletes	≈ 102 – M and F	Review of medical records	NA	3 years	X-ray or BS	2.9%†#
Johnson et al. 1994[18]	PC	Collegiate athletes	28 – F 60 – M	Monitoring	NA	2 years	X-ray or BS	3.6% – F 0% – M
Hickey et al. 1997[20]	CS	Elite: holders of scholarship	39 – F	Review of medical records	NA	5 years	NS	6.8%†
Swimming								
Goldberg and Pecora 1994[17]	CS	Collegiate athletes	≈ 225 – M and F	Review of medical records	NA	3 years	X-ray or BS	1.3%†#
Johnson et al. 1994[18]	PC	Collegiate athletes	34 – F 50 – M	Monitoring	NA	2 years	X-ray or BS	0% – F 0% – M

Notes: † Annual incidence. # Stress-fracture rates expressed as case rates: number of stress fractures per 100 athletes. M = Males. F = Females. NS = Not stated. NA = Not applicable. CC = Case–control. CS = Case series. HC = Historical cohort. PC = Prospective cohort. XS = Cross-sectional. BS = Bone scan. CT = Computed tomography. Hx = History.
Source: Adapted and reproduced, with permission, from Bennell KL, Brukner PD. Epidemiology and site-specificity of stress fractures. Clinics in Sports Medicine *1997; 16: 179–196.*

Table 2.2 Percentage of annual stress-fracture incidence: A comparison of various collegiate athletes in studies by Johnson et al.[18] and Goldberg and Pecora[17]

Sport	Johnson et al.[18]		Goldberg and Pecora[17] (%)†
	Men (%)	Women (%)	
Track	9.7	31.1	3.7
Crew	2.4	8.2	2.2
Lacrosse	4.3	3.1	2.7
Basketball	0	3.6	2.9
Football	1.1	NS	0.8
Soccer	0	2.6	2.0
Softball	NS	0	6.3
Swimming	0	0	1.3
Baseball	0	NS	2.6
Field hockey	NS	0	2.2
Tennis	0	0	2.8
Fencing	0	0	1.9
Volleyball	NS	0	2.4

Notes: † Approximate values, because denominator data were estimates. NS = Not studied.
In the study by Johnson et al.,[18] participant case rates were equivalent.
In the study by Goldberg and Pecora,[17] figures provided are case rates.

cohort study in order to investigate sports-related injuries in 914 collegiate male and female athletes. In total, thirty-four stress fractures were diagnosed by way of X-ray or bone scan (the same criteria used by Goldberg and Pecora[17]) over the study period. In males, the annual rate of stress-fracture incidence (expressed as a participant rate) was highest for track (9.7%), followed by lacrosse (4.3%), crew (2.4%), and American football (1.1%). No male athletes involved in baseball, basketball, fencing, golf, soccer, or tennis sustained a stress fracture. For women, the incidence rate for stress fracture was highest for track (31.1%), followed by crew (8.2%), basketball (3.6%), lacrosse (3.1%), and soccer (2.6%). No female athletes in fencing, field hockey, golf, softball, tennis, or volleyball sustained a stress fracture.

Although these two studies enable the sports to be ranked according to stress-fracture incidence, it must be remembered that neither study expressed incidence relative to exposure. It is possible that if training and playing hours were taken into account the stress-fracture risk may in fact be quite different from what has been reported. This should be kept in mind when likelihood of stress fracture is being compared in various sports. For example, if track athletes train and compete for many more hours than athletes do in other sports, the stress-fracture risk among track athletes could be lower if rates were expressed according to hours of participation.

RUNNING

Stress fractures seem to be a common injury in runners. This may be because of the continuous, repetitive muscular activity as well as the gravitational forces that result from ground impact. In one of the collegiate studies previously discussed,[18] both male and female track athletes had the highest stress-fracture incidence compared with athletes from other sports. In a prospective cohort study of ninety-five track and field athletes whose age ranged from seventeen to twenty-six years and who competed at club, state or national level, the annual participant stress-fracture rate (confirmed on bone scan and on X-ray or CT [computed-tomography] scan) was approximately 20% for both men and women.[5] When expressed as a case rate, the figure was even higher: 25% for men, and 30% for women. This is one of a limited number of athlete studies that also express stress-fracture incidence in terms of exposure. Results showed an overall rate of 0.70 stress fractures per 1000 training hours. To put this into perspective, were a group of ten athletes to train for ten hours per week, one athlete would be likely to develop a stress fracture after approximately fourteen weeks.

Studies in which self-administered questionnaires were used (with a known propensity for bias in recall and sampling) have found that 13% to 52% of female runners have had a history of stress fracture. The lowest frequency was found in a study that included recreational as well as competitive runners.[12] The very high participant rate of 52% (case rate of 85%) reported in female track and field athletes[19] may partly reflect sampling bias. In this study, subjects were recruited for a larger project in which risk factors for stress fractures were investigated. Athletes who had a history of stress fractures may have been more likely to respond to project advertising than were athletes who had never sustained a stress fracture.

Of 257 triathletes completing the Seafair Triathlon (a 1 kilometer swim, a 28 kilometer cycle, and a 10 kilometer run), 3.4% of women and 3.5% of men reported developing a stress fracture in the preceding year.[10] In all cases, the cause of injury was related to running, not swimming or cycling. However, because the rate of response to the questionnaire was low (45%), the results may not be representative of all competitors. Furthermore, the cohort comprised both elite and beginner triathletes, and it is possible that stress-fracture rates would be higher in one group than the other.

Despite the literature's shortcomings, stress fractures seem to be relatively frequent in running and in sports in which running forms a major component. Clinicians should therefore have a high index of suspicion for stress fracture when patients involved in these activities present with overuse pain in a lower limb.

BALLET DANCING

Although ballet studies to date have been mainly cross-sectional or case control in design, stress fractures also seem to be a relatively common injury in female dancers. In a survey of forty-five female classical-ballet dancers

approximately twenty years of age, 22% had sustained a stress fracture in the past year.[13] Using self-administered questionnaires, professional female dancers reported lifetime stress-fracture frequencies of 31.5%[15] and 45.0%.[8] When expressed as case rates, these figures were even higher: 50.0% and 67.5%, respectively. Stress-fracture rates for male dancers are lacking in the literature.

FIGURE SKATING

A self-administered questionnaire was used for eliciting information about stress-fracture history in forty-two male and female elite skaters.[14] Twenty-one percent of the skaters reported a history of stress fracture, although the definition of stress fracture was not specified. To our knowledge, this is the only study that has provided frequency of stress fractures in figure skaters.

GYMNASTICS

For elite gymnasts training at the Australian Institute of Sport over a ten-year period, stress-fracture case rates obtained through a review of medical records were 27.0% for females and 14.3% for males.[16] However, at a United States university, in male and female collegiate gymnastics in which approximately twelve participants were involved per year, only one stress fracture was sustained over a three-year period.[17] Greater volume and intensity of training may account for the greater number of stress fractures seen at the elite level compared with the collegiate level.

CREW

Rowing is an activity particularly associated with development of rib stress fractures. This may be related to bending stresses applied to the ribs by serratus anterior, latissimus dorsi and the rhomboids during the drive and catch phases of the rowing stroke. The annual rate of stress-fracture cases in collegiate crew members, obtained retrospectively by way of a review of medical records, was 3.3%.[17] The fractures were confined to the ribs.

Johnson et al.[18] prospectively reported that the average annual rate of collegiate rowers who had a stress fracture was 2.4% in men and 8.2% in women, although it is not clear what percentage of the fractures were located in the ribs. Two Australian studies of elite rowers have also reported stress-fracture rates. In a cohort of forty female elite rowers, three rib stress fractures were sustained over a four-year period.[11] In a ten-year review of 172 scholarship holders at the Australian Institute of Sport, there were fifteen rib stress fractures in eighty-four women: a case rate of 17.9%, and three stress fractures (two in the ribs and one in the ulna) in 88 men: 3.4%.[6] These figures are lower than those of the other studies, particularly when expressed according to the number of scholarship months. For women, there was one stress fracture per 103 months on scholarship, and for men there was one stress fracture per 548 months on scholarship. Despite the fact that stress fractures are relatively uncommon in rowers, a rib stress fracture should be considered in rowers who present with overuse thoracic pain.

BASKETBALL

The jumping, landing, and twisting components of basketball would be expected to subject the lower limb to relatively high-magnitude forces. In male and female collegiate basketballers combined, the average annual incidence of stress fractures was found to be 2.9%.[17] In females specifically, the average annual incidence has been reported as being 3.6% at collegiate level,[18] and 6.8% at elite level.[20] By comparison, none of the male collegiate basketballers in the study by Johnson et al.[18] sustained a fracture.

SWIMMING

Stress fractures do not seem to be a common injury in swimmers. None of the collegiate swimmers in the prospective cohort study of Johnson et al.[18] developed a stress fracture. Although another collegiate study did report an approximate 1.3% annual incidence of stress fractures in swimmers,[17] it is clear neither where the stress fractures were located nor whether they were caused by swimming or by other activities such as weight training or running, which often form part of a swimmer's training regimen.

Stress-fracture rates in the military

There are numerous studies in which stress-fracture rates in initial-entry, basic-training military populations are reported, and most use prospective cohort designs and large sample sizes[22–41] (Table 2.3). In male recruits, the reported stress-fracture participant and case rates range from 0.9% to 31% and from 0.2% to 62%, respectively. This variation is likely to reflect a number of factors, including recruits' type (Army, Airforce, or Marines), sex and age; the length (ranging from six to twenty-five weeks) and type of basic training; the country involved (most studies involve United States or Israeli recruits); the diagnostic criteria for stress fracture; and the method of injury tracking (active versus passive). For example, passive injury tracking leads to an underestimate of stress-fracture incidence. Beck et al.[36] reported an incidence of 3.7% using passive tracking of male recruits. However, active follow-up indicated that the actual stress-fracture rate was 6.2%; in other words, the self-reported stress-fracture rate under-reports the actual rate by approximately 40%.

Although rates for male United States recruits are less than 10% and most are approximately 1% to 3%, in two studies that involved the Israeli army the reported participant incidence rates were 31%[26] and 24%.[34] The researchers attributed the higher incidence to several factors, including meticulous follow-up (active monitoring), a high index of suspicion, and use

Table 2.3 Military studies in which stress-fracture incidence has been reported during basic training, expressed as a participant rate unless otherwise indicated

Reference	Study design	Population	Subjects	Observation period (weeks)	Diagnosis of stress fracture	Stress-fracture rate	
Protzman 1977[22]	PC	United States Army	102 – F 1228 – M	8	X-ray	9.8% – F# 1.0% – M#	
Reinker and Ozburne 1979[23]	HC	United States Army	NS – F 1198 – M	8	NS	2.2% – F# 0.8% – M#	
Kowal et al. 1980[24]	PC	United States Army	327 – F	8	X-ray	21.0%#	
Brudvig et al. 1983[25]	HC	United States Army and Marine	4422 – F 1600 – M	8	X-ray or BS	4.0%# 1.0%#	3.4% – F 0.9% – M
Milgrom et al. 1985[26]	PC	Israeli Army	295 – M	14	BS	62.0%#	31.0%
Jones et al. 1989[27]	PC	United States Army	186 – F 124 – M	8	NS	13.9% – F# 3.2% – M#	
Jones et al. 1989[27]	PC	United States Army	323 – M	13	NS	2.2%#	
Montgomery et al. 1989[28]	PC	United States Navy Sea, Air, and Land	505 – M	8	CE	6.3%	
Pester and Smith 1992[29]	PC	United States Army	33,059 – F 76,237 – M	8	X-ray or BS	1.1% – F 0.9% – M	
Taimela et al. 1992[30]	CT	Finnish Army	823 – M	12	X-ray	2.7%#	
Jones et al. 1993[31]	PC	United States Army	186 – F 124 – M	8	NS	12.3% – F# 2.4% – M#	
Jones et al. 1993[32]	PC	United States Army	303 – M	12	NS	3.0%#	
Jordaan and Schwellnus 1994[33]	PC	South African Army	1261 – M	9	X-ray	1.2%# 1.8 per 1000 training hours	
Milgrom et al. 1994[34]	CT	Israeli Army	783 – M	14	X-ray or BS	24.0%	

Table 2.3 continues.

Table 2.3 *continued*

Reference	Study design	Population	Subjects	Observation period (weeks)	Diagnosis of stress fracture	Stress-fracture rate
Shwayhat et al. 1994[35]	PC	United States Navy Sea, Air, and Land	224 – M	25	NS	6.7%#
Beck et al. 1996[36]	PC	United States Marine	626 – M	12	X-ray	4.3%# 3.7%
Cowan et al. 1996[37]	PC	United States Infantry	294 – M	12	NS	5.0%
Heir and Glomsaker 1996[38]	PC	Norwegian Army, Airforce, and Navy	6488 – M	6–10	NS	0.2%#
Bijur et al. 1997[39]	PC	United States Army	85 – F 473 – M	6	NS	15.0% – F 2.3% – M
Rudzki 1997[40]	CT	Australian Army	180 – M	12	NS	1.1%
Winfield et al. 1997[41]	PC	United States Navy	101 – F NS – M	10	X-ray or BS	11.5% – F 7.9% – M

Notes: # Stress-fracture rates, expressed as case rates: number of stress fractures per 100 recruits × 100. M = Males. F = Females. NS = Not stated. PC = Prospective cohort. HC = Historical cohort. CT = Clinical trial. BS = Bone scan. CE = Clinical examination.

of the isotope bone scan for diagnosis. Asymptomatic areas of uptake on bone scan were classified as stress fractures in the Israeli studies, and this is likely to overinflate the numbers reported; on the other hand, the United States military relies more heavily on radiographic diagnosis, which is less sensitive. Were the Israeli data to be adjusted using criteria used in United States studies, the stress-fracture rate would be approximately 6%, a figure that is more consistent with United States rates.[27] Recognition of the problem of stress fractures in particular and of overuse injuries in general has led to implementation of various preventive strategies. However, stress-fracture rates reported in more-recent United States military studies suggest that stress

fractures are a common problem for military personnel.

Stress-fracture rates in female military recruits undergoing basic training seem to be much higher than in males: they range from 1.1% to 21.0% (Table 2.3). This finding was recently the subject of a United States Army investigation.[42] What was found was that women report stress-induced injuries earlier than their male counterparts do in basic training, enter having a lower fitness level, are exposed to changes in stride length during coed marching, and engage in unique patterns of exercise that differ from the ones that male recruits engage in (for example dropping to the knees during push-ups). It is apparent that attention has to be paid to reducing stress-fracture incidence in female military recruits.

Stress-fracture recurrence rates

Clinically, stress-fracture recurrence is common. In a cross-sectional study of female track and field athletes, half of the athletes who reported a stress-fracture history had been treated for a stress fracture more than once.[19] When male and female track and field athletes were followed prospectively for one year, 60% of the ones who sustained a stress fracture had a previous stress-fracture history,[5] and the recurrence rate was 12.6%. In another study, a large number of male military recruits were followed for a minimum of one year after basic training.[43] The recurrence rate of stress fractures at a different site in recruits who had sustained a stress fracture during basic training was 10.6%. In the control group of sixty recruits who did not develop a stress fracture during basic training, stress-fracture incidence after basic training was only 1.7%.

It seems that people who have sustained a stress fracture in the past are at greater risk of developing a stress fracture at another site than are people who have never sustained a stress fracture. This may indicate persistence of risk factors in these people. From a clinical perspective, a history of stress fracture can be used as a marker for identifying people prone to stress fracture, thereby enabling preventive programs to be directed appropriately. It also emphasizes the necessity that stress-fracture treatment include strategies for minimizing the likelihood of another fracture.

Stress-fracture rates in various age groups

Although it is conceivable that stress-fracture rates vary with age, whether or not the rates increase or decrease with age is controversial. Bone density definitely decreases with age, and because of this, in older individuals, bone's ability to withstand repetitive loading could be reduced. On the other hand, children and adolescents may be at greater risk, because their bones are continuing to grow and have yet to reach their peak mass and strength. It is also possible that people who are likely to sustain a stress fracture change activities as they age. If they select themselves out of activities that may be more likely to produce a stress fracture, bias may be introduced.

Military studies enable stress-fracture rates to be compared in individuals of varying age who are engaged in identical or similar training programs. However, the age range is relatively narrow and in most cases is confined to early adulthood. In a historical cohort study of 20,422 military recruits, a review of clinical records found that stress-fracture incidence increased from 1.3% for 17- to 22-year-old Army recruits to 2.3% for 23- to 28-year-olds and to 5.0% for 29- to 34-year-olds.[25] The relative stress-fracture risk for the oldest age group compared with the youngest age group was 3.9. In the recruits who were more than thirty-five years of age, the incidence was 2.4%, but the group numbers were small and therefore considered to be unreliable. This higher stress-fracture risk because of age was also seen when men and women were evaluated separately (Fig. 2.1). Similar results have been reported in prospective cohort studies. Even when pre-training physical-activity levels were adjusted for recruits who were more than 21 years of age (of the 934 trainees in the group, only 37 were older than 25), these recruits had a relative stress-fracture risk of 1.7 (95% confidence intervals: 0.92, 3.21) compared with recruits who were 18 to 20 years old.[44]

Conversely, two other studies have found that younger recruits are more likely to develop stress fractures than are older recruits.[34,41] In female Marine trainees, the stress-fracture incidence rate was 17% in trainees who were less than 23 years old but only 2% in trainees who were more than 23 years of age.[41] Although the researchers claimed that this difference was statistically significant, the *P* value was given as 0.09, which

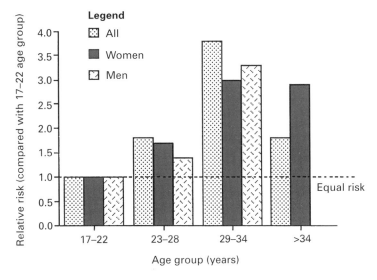

Fig. 2.1

Calculated relative risk of stress fractures over an eight-week army basic-training program for men ($n = 16{,}000$) and women ($n = 4422$) for each age group versus the youngest in Brudvig et al.[25] (Source: Adapted and reproduced, with permission, from Jones BH, Harris JM, Vinyh TN, Rubin C. Exercise-induced stress fractures and stress reactions of bone: epidemiology, etiology, and classification. *Exercise and Sport Sciences Reviews* 1989; 17: 379–422.)

in most other studies would not be considered to be a significant difference.

In a prospective study by Milgrom *et al.*[34] among male Israeli Army recruits, it was also reported that recruits who had a stress fracture were significantly younger than the recruits who did not, but the mean difference was small: approximately one month (18.58 years versus 18.70 years). Multivariate statistical analysis revealed that for each year of increase in age from 17 to 26 years, risk of stress fracture at all sites decreased by 28%. However, of the 783 recruits, only 26 were more than 19 years of age. The statistical results would therefore seem to be questionable, particularly for the post-teenage years. The other studies in which an increasing stress-fracture risk was found with increasing age had a greater spread of ages, and their results were analyzed differently by grouping ages together into categories. Although it is possible that within the seventeen-to-nineteen age range there is a decreasing risk for fracture, the risk may be less than that for people in the early- to-mid-twenties age range.

Whether or not age is a risk factor for stress fractures in athletes is not known. The difficulty

with reference to athletes lies in quantifying the amount and intensity of activity in populations of varying ages in order to enable an accurate comparison to be made of stress-fracture rates.[45] If differences in rates are found, they may simply be because of differences in exposure to physical activity, not because of age-related factors.

One case series of 1407 patients presenting to a sports-medicine center found that a greater percentage of injuries comprised stress fractures or periostitis in the 'younger' group (mean age of thirty years) than in the 'older' group (mean age of fifty-seven years).[46] However, because of the study design, it is not known whether or not this reflects selection of individuals in the older group who were stress-fracture resistant, modification of training regimens in order to reduce musculoskeletal stress, or an independent age effect on stress-fracture development.

Discrepancies exist in results obtained from military studies, whereby some have found an increase in stress-fracture risk with increasing age from the late teens to the mid-thirties and others have found a decreasing risk. At this stage, the athletics literature does not provide enough evidence for evaluating an age effect.

Stress-fracture rates in various ethnic groups

Generally, military studies suggest that risk for stress fractures is greater for both male and female Caucasians than for other racial groups, including Afro-Americans, Hispanics and Ethiopians[25,34,44] (Table 2.4). For White male recruits compared with African-Americans, relative stress-fracture risk was 4.7. This risk was even more pronounced for White female recruits: 8.5.[25] Similarly, Gardner *et al.*[44] showed that the stress-fracture risk for White

male Marines was 2.5 times higher than that for all other racial groups combined. The incidence rate was 1.56% for Whites, 0.60% for Blacks, and 0.67% for Hispanics. In the Israeli Army, there was a significant difference in stress-fracture incidence when Ethiopian recruits were compared with both Israeli-born and non-Israeli-born recruits. None of the Ethiopians sustained a stress fracture, in contrast to 24.8% of the other racial groups. Although in one prospective cohort study among 101 female Marine Corp recruits no significant difference in stress-fracture rates was reported between three racial groups (Whites, Black, and Others), the numbers in the non-White groups were small, and only nine stress fractures were sustained overall.[41]

Table 2.4 *Studies in which the rates and relative risk of stress fractures have been researched: a comparison of Caucasians (C) and Blacks (B). All rates are expressed as a participant rate unless otherwise indicated*

Reference	Population	Study design	Number C	Number B	Stress-fracture rate C	Stress-fracture rate B	Relative risk C versus B
Men							
Brudvig *et al.* 1983 (25)	Military	HC	NS	NS	1.1%	0.2%	4.7*
Gardner *et al.* 1988 (44)†	Military	CT	2050	975	1.6%#	0.7%#	2.3*
Milgrom *et al.* 1994 (34)	Military	CT	765	18	24.8%	0%	24.8*
Women							
Brudvig *et al.* 1983 (25)	Military	HC	NS	NS	11.8%	1.4%	8.5*
Barrow and Saha 1988 (9)	Athletes	XS	220	12	39.0%	17.0%	2.3

*Notes: * Statistically significant difference between races. # Stress-fracture rates, expressed as case rates: number of stress fractures per 100 recruits. † Blacks include all racial and ethnic groups other than Caucasians. NS = Not stated. PC = Prospective cohort. HC = Historical cohort. XS = Cross-sectional. CT = Clinical trial.*
Source: Adapted and reproduced, with permission, from Bennell KL, Brukner PD. Epidemiology and site-specificity of stress fractures. Clinics in Sports Medicine 1997; 179–196.

In the only athlete study in which stress-fracture rates were compared between racial groups, a cross-sectional design was used, the questionnaire response rate was only 24%, and again the number of African-Americans was small.[9] However, despite these limitations, a higher frequency of stress-fracture history was found in Caucasians: it was two times that in African-Americans.

Although the literature strongly suggests that Blacks and Hispanics are less likely to develop stress fractures, the reasons for this are not clear. Although it has been surmised that in these racial groups higher bone density and larger bones[47,48] may offer protection from stress fracture, none of the studies has included either bone mass or bone geometry as covariates during statistical analysis in order to evaluate the independent effects of ethnicity. Other suggested explanations include differences in biomechanic features such as foot type and lower limb alignment, or in anthropometric features such as amount of lean mass.[49]

Stress-fracture rates in men and women

It is commonly believed that women are at higher risk of developing stress fractures. Data from military populations lend credence to this viewpoint, but data from athletics studies are contradictory. Studies in which stress-fracture rates in women and men are directly compared are shown in Fig. 2.2. These studies consistently show that female recruits have greater risk of stress fracture, and that relative risks range from 1.2 to 10.0.[22,23,25,27,29,31,39,41] This increased risk persists even when training loads are applied gradually to a moderate level,

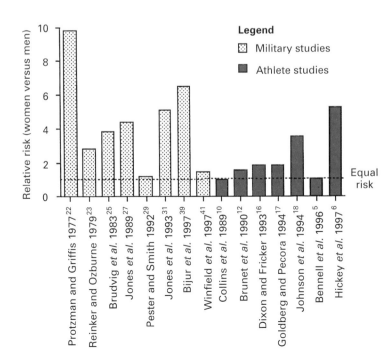

Fig. 2.2

Relative risk of stress fracture for women, compared with the risk for men, from military and athlete studies in which stress-fracture rates can be directly compared. (Source: Adapted and reproduced, with permission, from Bennell KL, Brukner PD. Epidemiology and site-specificity of stress fractures. *Clinics in Sports Medicine* 1997; 16: 179–196.)

and when age and race are taken into consideration.

As mentioned previously, this finding has been the subject of a recent investigation by the United States Army, particularly for determining whether bone density or dietary factors were contributory.[42] The report's conclusions are that a number of factors contribute to the gender-rate differential, including injury-reporting differences, fitness levels at the time of entry to basic training (higher in men), and biomechanic factors related to stride length and unique activities such as dropping to the knees during push-up drills. The relative importance of each factor, and the possibility that differences in diet and bone density are contributing factors, remain the subject of other research.

By contrast, it is less clear whether or not a sex difference exists in stress fracture rates in civilian populations[5,6,10,12,16–18] (Fig. 2.2). In some studies an increased risk of fracture in female athletes, up to 5.3 times that of men, has been reported. The greatest relative risk was found in elite rowers. Conversely, in other studies, including a prospective cohort study, the researchers have failed to find a difference between men and women in rates of stress-fracture incidence. Unlike the military, in which the amount and intensity of basic training are rigidly controlled, in most civilian studies it is difficult to assume that there is equivalence of training between the sexes. Because training is rigidly controlled in the military, opportunity for training-load self-selection is eliminated, and may in fact be the main reason for the reported gender-rate difference.

In one athlete study, in order to account for possible training differences between the sexes, incidence rates were expressed in terms of training hours.[5] No significant differences were found between incidence rates: women sustained 0.86 stress fractures per 1000 training hours, compared with 0.54 for men. Even so, expressing incidence in this way does not guarantee there

will be equivalence of training between the sexes, because differences in intensity and type of training could exist.

From military data, it is clear that female trainees are more likely to develop a stress fracture during basic training. Anecdotally, although female athletes also seem to be at greater risk, this has not been conclusively supported by scientific findings. This may be partly related to methodology issues, especially to the difficulty involved in controlling confounding factors such as type, volume, and intensity of training.

Frequency of stress fractures relative to other overuse injuries

In numerous case series, it has been reported that of all injuries sustained by athlete populations, stress fractures account for between 0.7% and 15.6%.[16,50–55] In a recent study of 2429 injuries presenting to an Australian sports-medicine center, stress fractures accounted for 3.6%.[56] In studies in which only runners were investigated, the relative frequency is higher: it ranges from 6.0% to 15.6%. In track and field athletes, stress fractures accounted for a large percentage of overuse injuries: 34.2% in women and 24.4% in men, as reported in one study,[57] and 42.0% for men and women combined, as reported in another.[50] In elite gymnasts, stress fractures accounted for 18.3% of overuse injuries in women, and 9.2% in men.[16] The variation in results probably reflects differences in the composition of each case series. Composition is affected by factors such as referral patterns; case loads; area of practise; and demographics and participation patterns of patients in the clinics, including training intensity, type of sport, and percentage of elite versus recreational athletes.

Site distribution of stress fractures

ATHLETE POPULATIONS

Although stress fractures are most common in lower-extremity bones, they also occur in non-weightbearing bones, including the ribs and upper limbs. In numerous studies, the anatomic distribution of series of stress fractures has been reported[5,9,15,17,18,50,52–54,58–65] (Table 2.5). Great variation exists in the absolute percentage of stress fractures reported at each bony site, but the most common sites seem to be the tibia, metatarsals, and fibula.

A number of factors may influence reported distributions of stress fractures, including the patient's gender, age, and type and level of activity, as well as method of stress-fracture diagnosis. For example, tarsal navicular stress fractures give rise to subtle clinical findings, are often missed in differential diagnosis of foot and ankle pain, and are rarely evident on radiographs. They will therefore be under-reported compared with stress fractures such as ones that occur in the metatarsals, for which clinical and radiographic diagnoses are more straightforward.

In his excellent 1975 monograph, Devas reported that when clinical examination and plain radiography are used for diagnosing stress fractures, the fibula, second metatarsal, and calcaneus are commonly affected.[66] Recent case reports of stress fractures at previously unreported sites such as the ulnar diaphysis,[67] patella,[68] and neck of the seventh and eighth ribs[69] may reflect development of more-sensitive imaging techniques such as magnetic resonance imaging (MRI) and the triple-phase isotope bone scan, as well as increased awareness of stress fractures.

Specific stress-fracture sites are more commonly associated with specific sports. This is not to say that occurrence of stress fractures in these sites in these sports is exclusive, but that the sites' relative frequency compared with other sites is greater. This probably reflects the loads applied to the skeleton during various activities. In a series of 180 stress fractures, the percentage distribution of sports among the five most common sites is set out in Table 2.6.[70] Dancers sustained the largest number of metatarsal stress fractures, track and distance runners sustained the most tibial stress fractures, and distance runners and dancers incurred the most fibular stress fractures. Navicular stress fractures were by far the most common fracture among track athletes. Fractures of the pars interarticularis were seen among athletes in field events, racket sports, cricket, dancing, and basketball. Other sports associated with specific stress fractures are rowing and golf (rib stress fractures), pitching (humeral fractures), and gymnastics (pars fractures).

Although various sports are more commonly associated with specific stress fractures (Table 2.7), virtually any stress fracture can occur in almost any sport. Recognizing that no studies exist in which the relationship between a specific sport or activity and a specific stress-fracture site is clearly defined, the site distribution relative to sport participation is only partially helpful for the clinician, who must have a high index of suspicion for stress fracture in virtually every type of physical activity.

Conditioned athletes may sustain stress fractures at sites different from the ones in people unaccustomed to activity. In a series of 368 fractures, competitive athletes had more tibial stress fractures, whereas recreational athletes had more metatarsal and pelvic-bone fractures.[52,60] It has also been reported that females sustain more metatarsal,[52,60] pelvic,[60] and navicular stress fractures,[18] although this is not always borne out by clinical experience. Age differences may play a part: Matheson *et al.*[61] found more femoral and tarsal stress fractures in older athletes, and more tibial and fibular stress fractures in younger athletes. However, interaction between age and stress-fracture site

Table 2.5 Anatomic distribution of stress fractures in athletes, expressed as a percentage of the total number of stress fractures in each series

Reference	Sport	Number of stress fractures in series	Diagnosis of stress fracture	Tibia (%)	Fibula (%)	Metatarsal (%)	Navicular (%)	Femur (%)	Pelvis (%)
Brubaker and James 1974[50]	Runners	17	NS	41.2	17.6	29.4	5.9	0	0
Orava 1980[52]	Variety	200	X-ray plus or instead of BS	53.5	12.5	18.0	2.0	6.0	1.5
Pagliano and Jackson 1980[53]	Runners	99	Self-reporting	20.2	15.2	37.4	NS	NS	NS
Taunton et al. 1981[58]	Runners	62	X-ray or BS	55.0	11.3	16.1	3.2	6.5	0
Clement et al. 1981[54]	Runners	87	NS	57.5	9.2	20.7	3.4	4.6	0
Sullivan et al. 1984[59]	Runners	57	X-ray or BS	43.9	21.0	14.0	0	3.5	10.5
Hulkko and Orava 1987[60]	Variety	368	X-ray plus or instead of BS	49.5	12.0	19.8	2.5	6.3	1.9
Matheson et al. 1987[61]	Variety	320	BS	49.1	6.6	8.8	NS	7.2	1.6
Barrow and Saha 1988[9]	Runners	140	Self-reporting	63.0	9.0	21.0	0.7	4.0	1.4
Courtenay and Bowers 1990[62]	Variety	108	X-ray or BS	38.0	29.6	18.5	4.6	2.8	0.9
Ha et al. 1991[63]	Variety	169	X-ray or BS	31.5	10.7	7.1	4.7	12.5	4.1
Benazzo et al. 1992[64]	Track and field	49	X-ray, CT, or BS	26.5	12.2	14.3	28.6	0	0
Kadel et al. 1992[15]	Ballet	27	Self-reporting	22.0	0	63.0	NS	4.0	0
Goldberg and Pecora 1994[17]	Variety	58	X-ray or BS	18.9	12.1	25.9	NS	10.0	3.4
Johnson et al. 1994[18]	Variety	34	X-ray plus or instead of BS	38.2	0	20.6	11.8	23.5	0
Bennell et al. 1996[5]	Track and field	26	BS and CT	45.0	12.0	8.0	15.0	8.0	4.0
Brukner et al. 1996[65]	Variety	180	X-ray, CT, or BS	20.0	16.7	23.3	20.0	3.3	1.1
Hickey et al. 1997[20]	Basketball	22	NS	37.5	17.5	15.0	10.0	5.0	0

Notes: *BS = Bone scan. CT = Computed tomography. NS = Not stated.*
Source: *Adapted and reproduced, with permission, from Bennell KL, Brukner PD. Epidemiology and site-specificity of stress fractures.* Clinics in Sports Medicine *1997; 16: 179–196.*

Table 2.6 Percentage distribution of sports among the most common stress-fracture sites

Sport	Metatarsal (%) (n = 42)	Tibia (%) (n = 36)	Fibula (%) (n = 30)	Tarsal navicular (%) (n = 26)	Pars interarticularis (%) (n = 17)
Track	21.4	38.9	16.7	73.1	5.8
Jogging distance or running	11.9	41.7	26.7	3.8	0
Dance	42.9	2.8	23.3	0	17.6
Australian football	4.8	8.3	10.0	7.7	0
Racket sports	2.4	2.8	6.7	3.8	17.6
Field events	0	0	6.7	0	23.5
Rowing or canoeing	2.4	0	3.3	3.8	0
Triathlon	2.4	0	3.3	3.8	0
Basketball	2.4	0	0	3.8	11.8
Cricket	0	0	0	0	17.6
Aerobics	7.2	0	3.3	0	0
Field hockey	0	0	0	0	5.9
Rugby	0	2.8	0	0	0
Martial arts	2.4	0	0	0	0
Work related	0	0	0	0	5.9

Source: Adapted and reproduced, with permission, from Brukner P, Bradshaw C, Khan KM et al. Stress fractures: a review of 180 cases. Clinical Journal of Sport Medicine 1996; 6: 85.

was not confirmed in another large series.[60] Although specific individual characteristics may influence stress fractures' site distribution, their exact influence has not been clearly elucidated.

MILITARY RECRUITS

In military personnel, the site distribution of stress fractures has changed over the years, because running instead of marching has been emphasized, athletics shoes instead of combat boots have been worn, recruits' fitness level has been higher, and advances in imaging technology have been made. In original reports, injuries of the foot were mainly described, and most stress fractures were diagnosed as occurring in the metatarsals.[71,72] Even in the early 1990s, fractures of the foot were relatively more common than fractures in the lower limb, particularly in men.

For example, in a series of 1338 stress fractures that were sustained over a four-year period, the most common sites for male recruits were the metatarsals (66%), followed by the calcaneus (20%), and the lower leg (13%).[29] For women, the sites were the calcaneus (39%), the metatarsals (31%), and the lower leg (27%). In more-recent studies, a greater number of stress fractures in the leg have been found, particularly of the tibia; these results therefore more closely approximate the site characteristics observed in athlete populations. In 1261 South African recruits, out of fourteen stress fractures confirmed by way of X-ray, 71% were located in the tibial shaft, and only 21% were located in the metatarsals.[33] In a recent prospective study of 626 male United States Marine Corps recruits,

Table 2.7 Sports and activities commonly associated with various stress-fracture sites

Stress-fracture site	Sport or activity
Coracoid process of scapula	Trap shooting
Scapula	Running with hand-held weights
Humerus	Throwing and racket sports
Olecranon	Throwing and pitching
Ulna	Racket sports (especially tennis), gymnastics, volleyball, swimming, softball, and wheelchair sports
Ribs – first	Throwing and pitching
Ribs – second to tenth	Rowing and kayaking
Pars interarticularis	Gymnastics, ballet, cricket fast bowling, volleyball, and springboard diving
Pubic ramus	Distance running and ballet
Femur – neck	Distance running, jumping, and ballet
Femur – shaft	Distance running
Patella	Running and hurdling
Tibia – plateau	Running
Tibia – shaft	Running and ballet
Fibula	Running, aerobics, race-walking, and ballet
Medial malleolus	Basketball and running
Calcaneus	Long-distance military marching
Talus	Pole vaulting
Navicular	Sprinting, middle-distance running, hurdling, long or triple jumping, and football
Metatarsal – general	Running, ballet, and marching
Metatarsal – base second	Ballet
Metatarsal – fifth	Tennis and ballet
Sesamoid bones of foot	Running, ballet, basketball, and skating

Source: Adapted and reproduced, with permission, from Brukner PD, Khan KM. Clinical Sports Medicine. *Sydney: McGraw-Hill, 1993: 17.*

27 stress fractures were sustained.[36] The most common site was the tibia (41%), followed by the metatarsals (26%), the femur (19%), and the tarsals (15%). These figures are similar to the ones reported by Winfield *et al.*[41] in terms of both the relative ranking and the absolute percentages. In women, the tibia was the most common site (50%), followed by the metatarsals (25%). In men, tibial and metatarsal stress fractures were equal in frequency (40%).

Stress-fracture morbidity

One way of assessing injury morbidity is to measure the resulting extent of disability. In their series of stress fractures in athletes, Hulkko and Orava[60] reported that 77% of the athletes had symptoms only during training whereas 13% had symptoms in everyday life. Loss of time from work was required in 10% of cases.

In the military, stress fractures can be evaluated according to the number of lost training days. In one study, stress fractures were responsible for the greatest number of training days lost as a result of injury (21.6 days lost per stress fracture).[33] Of the stress-fracture sites, the femoral-shaft fractures resulted in the most lost training days (forty-nine days per fracture).

In most other studies, stress-fracture morbidity is expressed as the time taken until recovery, and recovery is usually defined as full return to sport or activity. For example, Benazzo et al.[64] found a mean time of 4.4 months for return to sport, and showed that the figure was directly related to the time between symptom onset and establishment of a diagnosis. Conversely, Matheson et al.[61] reported a shorter mean recovery time of 12.8 weeks, but the range was from two to ninety-six weeks. However, unlike the Benazzo et al. study, no correlation was evident between the time to diagnosis and the time to recovery. Matheson et al. also found that tarsal stress fractures took the longest time, and femoral fractures the least. Mean recovery times reported in case series have varied, probably due to the subjectivity of return-to-sport criteria and to differences in distribution of stress-fracture sites. Because healing times are site dependent, morbidity should be evaluated separately for various stress-fracture sites.

In Table 2.8, the healing times are set out according to site in a series of 368 stress fractures in athletes.[60] It is evident that at some sites, such as the femoral neck, the sesamoids, and the middle third of the tibia, recovery usually took longer than two months. However, at other sites, such as the fibula and the metatarsals, recovery took less than two months. Most stress fractures usually heal uneventfully. In a follow-up (of unspecified duration) of fifty-one runners who had a stress fracture, 82% of the athletes were running symptom free, 16% had recurrent pain at the fracture site while running, and 2% ceased running because of recurrent pain.[59] Sixty-six recruits who had suffered a stress fracture during a prospective study were followed for a minimum of one year

Table 2.8 Percentage of stress fractures healed at various times in a case series of 368 stress fractures in athletes

Stress-fracture site	Healing period		
	2–4 weeks (%)	1–2 months (%)	>2 months (%)
Tibia			
Proximal third	0	43	57
Middle third	0	48	52
Distal third	0	53	47
Fibula	7	75	18
Metatarsals	20	57	23
Sesamoids	0	0	100
Femur			
Shaft	7	7	86
Neck	0	0	100
Pelvis	0	29	71
Olecranon	0	0	100

Source: Adapted and reproduced, with permission, from Hulkko A, Orava S. Stress fractures in athletes. International Journal of Sports Medicine *1987; 8: 221–226.*

after their basic training.[43] There was uneventful recovery in 47.0%, protracted recovery in 13.6%, recurrent stress fractures in new sites in 19.6%, intermittent bone pain that was not related to stress fracture in 16.7%, and chronic stress fracture in 3.0%.

Some sites are prone to delayed or nonunion, and people who have a stress fracture in one of them are more likely to be prevented from returning to their previous activity level. The sites include the anterior cortex of the tibia, and the tarsal navicular. For example, Khan et al.[73] found that in navicular stress fractures, 86% of patients who at first had treatment that involved non-weightbearing cast immobilization returned to their sport, compared with only 26% who continued weightbearing. Of the patients who were treated surgically, 73% were able to return to sport. These difficult fractures will be discussed in more detail in the chapters in which the specific regions are discussed.

SUMMARY

- Stress fractures are a common overuse injury in athletes and in military recruits who are undertaking basic training.
- Although there are a lack of well-conducted studies in which sound epidemiological principles are used to document stress fractures' incidence and prevalence rates in athletes, a number of important insights can be gleaned from the literature.
- The available data suggest that runners and ballet dancers are at relatively high risk for stress fractures.
- Although a gender difference in rates is evident in military populations, it is less evident in athletes.
- Other participant characteristics such as age and race may also influence stress-fracture risk.
- In athletes, the most common stress-fracture site is the tibia.
- Stress-fracture morbidity, expressed as the time until return to sport or activity, varies, depending on the site.
- For healing, a period of six to eight weeks is usually required. However, stress fractures at some sites, such as the navicular and the anterior tibial cortex, are often associated with protracted recovery and, in some cases, termination of sporting pursuits.

References

1. Walter SD, Sutton JR, McIntosh JM, Connolly C. The aetiology of sports injuries: a review of methodologies. *Sports Medicine* 1985; 2: 47–58.

2. Hennekens CH, Buring JE. *Epidemiology in Medicine*, 5th edn. Boston: Little, Brown and Company, 1987.

3. Meeuwisse WH. Athletic injury etiology: distinguishing between interaction and confounding. *Clinical Journal of Sport Medicine* 1994; 4: 171–175.

4. Caine CG, Caine DJ, Lindner KJ. The epidemiologic approach to sports injuries. In: Caine DJ, Caine CG, Lindner KJ, eds. *Epidemiology of Sports Injuries*. Champaign: Human Kinetics, 1996: 1–13.

5. Bennell KL, Malcolm SA, Thomas SA, Wark JD, Brukner PD. The incidence and distribution of stress fractures in competitive track and field athletes. *American Journal of Sports Medicine* 1996; 24: 211–217.

6. Hickey GJ, Fricker PA, McDonald WA. Injuries to elite rowers over a 10-yr period. *Medicine and Science in Sports and Exercise* 1997; 29: 1567–1572.

7. Lloyd T, Triantafyllou SJ, Baker ER *et al.* Women athletes with menstrual irregularity have increased musculoskeletal injuries. *Medicine and Science in Sports and Exercise* 1986; 18: 374–379.

8. Warren MP, Brooks-Gunn J, Hamilton LH, Warren LF, Hamilton WG. Scoliosis and fractures in young ballet dancers. *New England Journal of Medicine* 1986; 314: 1348–1353.

9. Barrow GW, Saha S. Menstrual irregularity and stress fractures in collegiate female distance runners. *American Journal of Sports Medicine* 1988; 16: 209–216.

10. Collins K, Wagner M, Peterson K, Storey M. Overuse injuries in triathletes: a study of the 1986 Seafair Triathlon. *American Journal of Sports Medicine* 1989; 17: 675–680.

11. Reid RA, Fricker PA, Kestermann O, Shakespear P. A profile of female rowers' injuries and illnesses at the Australian Institute of Sport. *Excel* 1989; 5: 17–20.

12. Brunet ME, Cook SD, Brinker MR, Dickinson JA. A survey of running injuries in 1505 competitive and recreational runners. *Journal of Sports Medicine and Physical Fitness* 1990; 30: 307–315.

13. Frusztajer NT, Dhuper S, Warren MP, Brooks-Gunn J, Fox RP. Nutrition and the incidence of stress fractures in ballet dancers. *American Journal of Clinical Nutrition* 1990; 51: 779–783.

14. Pecina M, Bojanic I, Dubravcic S. Stress fractures in figure skaters. *American Journal of Sports Medicine* 1990; 18: 277–279.

15. Kadel NJ, Teitz CC, Kronmal RA. Stress fractures in ballet dancers. *American Journal of Sports Medicine* 1992; 20: 445–449.

16. Dixon M, Fricker P. Injuries to elite gymnasts over 10 yr. *Medicine and Science in Sports and Exercise* 1993; 25: 1322–1329.

17 Goldberg B, Pecora C. Stress fractures: a risk of increased training in freshmen. *Physician and Sportsmedicine* 1994; 22: 68–78.

18 Johnson AW, Weiss CB, Wheeler DL. Stress fractures of the femoral shaft in athletes – more common than expected: a new clinical test. *American Journal of Sports Medicine* 1994; 22: 248–256.

19 Bennell KL, Malcolm SA, Thomas SA *et al.* Risk factors for stress fractures in female track-and-field athletes: a retrospective analysis. *Clinical Journal of Sport Medicine* 1995; 5: 229–235.

20 Hickey GJ, Fricker PA, McDonald WA. Injuries to young elite female basketball players over a six-year period. *Clinical Journal of Sport Medicine* 1997; 7: 252–256.

21 Nattiv A, Puffer JC, Green GA. Lifestyles and health risks of collegiate athletes – a multi-center study. *Clinical Journal of Sport Medicine* 1997; 7: 262–272.

22 Protzman RR, Griffis CC. Comparative stress fracture incidence in males and females in an equal training environment. *Athletic Training* 1977; 12: 126–130.

23 Reinker KA, Ozburne S. A comparison of male and female orthopaedic pathology in basic training. *Military Medicine* 1979; August: 532–536.

24 Kowal DM. Nature and causes of injuries in women resulting from an endurance training program. *American Journal of Sports Medicine* 1980; 8: 265–269.

25 Brudvig TJS, Gudger TD, Obermeyer L. Stress fractures in 295 trainees: a one-year study of incidence as related to age, sex, and race. *Military Medicine* 1983; 148: 666–667.

26 Milgrom C, Giladi M, Stein M *et al.* Stress fractures in military recruits: a prospective study showing an unusually high incidence. *Journal of Bone and Joint Surgery* 1985; 67-B: 732–735.

27 Jones H, Harris JM, Vinh TN, Rubin C. Exercise-induced stress fractures and stress reactions of bone: epidemiology, etiology, and classification. *Exercise and Sports Sciences Review* 1989; 17: 379–422.

28 Montgomery LC, Nelson FRT, Norton JP, Deuster FA. Orthopedic history and examination in the etiology of overuse injuries. *Medicine and Science in Sports and Exercise* 1989; 21: 237–243.

29 Pester S, Smith PC. Stress fractures in the lower extremities of soldiers in basic training. *Orthopaedic Review* 1992; 21: 297–303.

30 Taimela S, Kujala UM, Dahlstrom S, Koskinen S. Risk factors for stress fractures during physical training programs. *Clinical Journal of Sport Medicine* 1992; 2: 105–108.

31 Jones BH, Bovee MW, Harris JM, Cowan DN. Intrinsic risk factors for exercise-related injuries among male and female army trainees. *American Journal of Sports Medicine* 1993; 21: 705–710.

32 Jones BH, Cowan DN, Tomlinson JP *et al.* Epidemiology of injuries associated with physical training among young men in the army. *Medicine and Science in Sports and Exercise* 1993; 25: 197–203.

33 Jordaan G, Schwellnus MP. The incidence of overuse injuries in military recruits during basic military training. *Military Medicine* 1994; 159: 421–426.

34 Milgrom C, Finestone A, Shlamkovitch N *et al.* Youth is a risk factor for stress fracture: a study of 783 infantry recruits. *Journal of Bone and Joint Surgery* 1994; 76-B: 20–22.

35 Shwayhat AF, Linenger JM, Hofherr LK, Slymen DJ, Johnson CW. Profiles of exercise history and overuse injuries among United States navy sea, air, and land (SEAL) recruits. *American Journal of Sports Medicine* 1994; 22: 835–840.

36 Beck TJ, Ruff CB, Mourtada FA *et al.* Dual-energy x-ray absorptiometry derived structural geometry for stress fracture prediction in male U.S. Marine Corps recruits. *Journal of Bone and Mineral Research* 1996; 11: 645–653.

37 Cowan DN, Jones BH, Frykman PN *et al.* Lower limb morphology and risk of overuse injury among male infantry trainees. *Medicine and Science in Sports and Exercise* 1996; 28: 945–952.

38 Heir T, Glomsaker P. Epidemiology of musculoskeletal injuries among Norwegian conscripts undergoing basic military training. *Scandinavian Journal of Medicine and Science in Sports* 1996; 6: 186–191.

39 Bijur PE, Horodyski M, Egerton W *et al.* Comparison of injury during cadet basic training by gender. *Archives of Pediatric and Adolescent Medicine* 1997; 151: 456–461.

40 Rudzki SJ. Injuries in Australian army recruits. Part II: Location and cause of injuries seen in recruits. *Military Medicine* 1997; 162: 477–480.

41 Winfield AC, Bracker M, Moore J, Johnson CW. Risk factors associated with stress reactions in female marines. *Military Medicine* 1997; 162: 698–702.

42 Schneeman BO, Nesheim RO, Bilezikian JP *et al. Reducing Stress Fracture in Physically Active Military Women.* Subcommittee on Body Composition, Nutrition, and Health of Military Women; and Committee on Military Nutrition Research, Food and Nutrition Board, Institute of Medicine. Washington DC: National Academy Press, 1998.

43 Milgrom C, Giladi M, Chisin R, Dizian R. The long-term followup of soldiers with stress fractures. *American Journal of Sports Medicine* 1985; 13: 398–400.

44 Gardner LI, Dziados JE, Jones BH *et al.* Prevention of lower extremity stress fractures: a controlled trial of a shock absorbent insole. *American Journal of Public Health* 1988; 78: 1563–1567.

45 Burr DB. Bone, exercise, and stress fractures. *Exercise and Sport Sciences Reviews* 1997; 25: 171–194.

46 Matheson GO, Macintyre JG, Taunton JE, Clement DB, Lloyd-Smith R. Musculoskeletal injuries associated with physical activity in older adults. *Medicine and Science in Sports and Exercise* 1989; 21: 379–385.

47 Cohn SH, Abesamis C, Yasumura S *et al.* Comparative skeletal mass and radial bone mineral content in black and white women. *Metabolism* 1977; 26: 171–178.

48 Meyer SA, Saltzman CL, Albright JP. Stress fractures of the foot and leg. *Clinics in Sports Medicine* 1993; 12: 395–413.

49 Giladi M, Milgrom C, Stein M *et al.* The low arch: a protective factor in stress fractures. A prospective study of 295 military recruits. *Orthopaedic Review* 1985; 14: 709–712.

50 Brubaker CE, James SL. Injuries to runners. *Journal of Sports Medicine* 1974; 2: 189–198.

51 James SL, Bates BT, Osternig LR. Injuries to runners. *American Journal of Sports Medicine* 1978; 6: 40–49.

52 Orava S. Stress fractures. *British Journal of Sports Medicine* 1980; 14: 40–44.

53 Pagliano J, Jackson D. The ultimate study of running injuries. *Runners World* 1980; November: 42–50.

54 Clement DB, Taunton JE, Smart GW, McNicol KL. A survey of overuse running injuries. *Physician and Sportsmedicine* 1981; 9: 47–58.

55 Witman PA, Melvin M, Nicholas JA. Common problems seen in a metropolitan sports injury clinic. *Physician and Sportsmedicine* 1981; 9: 105–108.

56 Baquie P, Brukner P. Injuries presenting to an Australian Sports Medicine Centre: a 12-month study. *Clinical Journal of Sport Medicine* 1997; 7: 28–31.

57 Bennell KL, Crossley K. Musculoskeletal injuries in track and field: incidence, distribution and risk factors. *Australian Journal of Science and Medicine in Sport* 1996; 28: 69–75.

58 Taunton JE, Clement DB, Webber D. Lower extremity stress fractures in athletes. *Physician and Sportsmedicine* 1981; 9: 77–86.

59 Sullivan D, Warren RF, Pavlov H, Kelman G. Stress fractures in 51 runners. *Clinical Orthopaedics and Related Research* 1984; 187: 188–189.

60 Hulkko A, Orava S. Stress fractures in athletes. *International Journal of Sports Medicine* 1987; 8: 221–226.

61 Matheson GO, Clement DB, McKenzie DC *et al.* Stress fractures in athletes: a study of 320 cases. *American Journal of Sports Medicine* 1987; 15: 46–58.

62 Courtenay BG, Bowers DM. Stress fractures: clinical features and investigation. *Medical Journal of Australia* 1990; 153: 155–156.

63 Ha KI, Hahn SH, Chung M, Yang BK, Yi SR. A clinical study of stress fractures in sports activities. *Orthopaedics* 1991; 14: 1089–1095.

64 Benazzo F, Barnabei G, Ferrario A, Castelli C, Fischetto G. Stress fractures in track and field athletes. *Journal of Sports Traumatology and Related Research* 1992; 14: 51–65.

65 Brukner P, Bradshaw C, Khan K, White S. Stress fractures: a review of 180 cases. *Clinical Journal of Sport Medicine* 1996; 6: 85–89.

66 Devas M. *Stress Fractures.* Edinburgh: Churchill Livingstone, 1975.

67 Escher SA. Ulnar diaphyseal stress fracture in a bowler. *American Journal of Sports Medicine* 1997; 25: 412–413.

68 Mata SG, Grande MM, Overjero AH. Transverse stress fracture of the patella – a case report. *Clinical Journal of Sport Medicine* 1996; 6: 259–261.

69 Brukner P, Khan K. Stress fracture of the neck of the seventh and eighth ribs – a case report. *Clinical Journal of Sport Medicine* 1996; 6: 204–206.

70 Brukner PD, Bennell KL. Stress fractures in runners. *Journal of Back and Musculoskeletal Rehabilitation* 1995; 5: 341–351.

71 Carlson GD, Wertz RF. March fracture, including others than those of the foot. *Journal of Bone and Joint Surgery* 1944; 43: 48–54.

72 Hullinger CW. Insufficiency fracture of the calcaneus: similar to march fracture of the metatarsal. *Journal of Bone and Joint Surgery* 1944; 26: 751–757.

73 Khan KM, Fuller PJ, Brukner PD, Kearney C, Burry HC. Outcome of conservative and surgical management of navicular stress fracture in athletes. *American Journal of Sports Medicine* 1992; 20: 657–666.

Chapter 3

The risk factors for stress fractures

For sports-medicine practitioners, to prevent stress fractures is a major goal. In order to prevent injury, the causative factors and the mechanisms by which they interact have to be clearly understood. If practitioners have this knowledge, they can evaluate preventive measures (Fig. 3.1). In this chapter, the role of risk factors in stress-fracture pathogenesis is reviewed.

Interaction of risk factors

Risk factors for any injury may be classified as extrinsic (external) or intrinsic (internal). Extrinsic factors are characteristics of the environment in which the athlete participates, whereas intrinsic factors are characteristics of the athletes themselves. Injuries occur as a result of summation of various extrinsic and intrinsic factors at a given point in time.[1] For stress fractures, potential extrinsic risk factors include training methods and equipment, whereas intrinsic factors can be muscular, mechanical, hormonal or nutritional. The potential risk factors are set out in the following summary.

As well as a given risk factor's independent effects and its mechanism of contribution to bone injury, interactions between risk factors are possible,[2] as set out in Table 3.1.

SUMMARY POTENTIAL RISK FACTORS FOR STRESS FRACTURE

Intrinsic mechanical factors
- Bone-mineral density
- Bone geometry
- Skeletal alignment
- Body size and composition

Physiologic factors
- Bone turnover
- Muscle flexibility and joint range of motion
- Muscular strength and endurance

Nutritional factors
- Calcium intake
- Caloric intake and eating disorders
- Nutrient deficiencies

Hormonal factors
- Sex hormones
- Menarcheal age
- Other hormones

Physical training
- Physical fitness
- Volume of training
- Pace of training
- Intensity of training
- Recovery periods

Extrinsic mechanical factors
- Surface
- Footwear, insoles, and orthotics
- External loading

Other factors
- Genetic predisposition
- Psychological traits

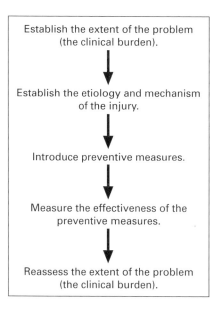

Fig. 3.1

Sports-injury prevention. The sequence includes first establishing the extent of the clinical burden (morbidity). This is followed by establishing the injury's pathophysiology and etiology, and includes identifying intrinsic and extrinsic risk factors and their relative importance. Next, preventive measures are evaluated for their effectiveness in reducing risk of injury. Finally, the measures' effect has to be evaluated by again assessing the clinical burden (the nature and extent of the problem).

In order to ascertain each risk factor's relative importance, following is a critical evaluation of the available literature. First, the issues that affect the validity of conclusions presented in studies of risk factors for stress fractures are briefly reviewed.

Methodology issues

STUDY DESIGN

Many issues are related to the rigor of clinical studies that affect the validity of the conclusions drawn from the studies; the type of design used, for example, has considerable impact. Much of the stress-fracture literature consists of case series that although useful for hypothesis generation cannot be used for determining a cause-and-effect relationship between a given risk factor and subsequent stress-fracture development. In order to best evaluate risk, information about the uninjured population is required. In any study in which only events are described, true comparisons cannot be made between injured and noninjured groups.

CROSS-SECTIONAL STUDIES, OR SURVEYS

These are a special type of study design in which comparisons can be made between injured and noninjured groups. A correlation can be drawn between a supposed risk factor and an injury. However, in this type of study design a cause-and-effect relationship cannot be established, because both the risk factor and the injury are documented at the same point in time. For example, if a difference in flexibility (risk factor) is found between runners some of whom have and some of whom do not have a lower-extremity stress fracture, it is not possible to know whether flexibility contributed to the injury's development or whether flexibility changed because of the injury. This illustrates the critical distinction between correlation and causation.

ANALYTIC STUDIES

In these studies, an attempt is made to understand events and to test hypotheses. Typically, they are experimental designs (clinical trials) and observational designs that are analytic in nature (cohort and case-control studies), and involve use of a comparison or control group in order to study differences in the variable under study. Also, the intervention or risk factor clearly precedes the outcome's development (injury), so a cause-and-effect relationship can be established.[2] Study-design knowledge is important for clinicians, because it enables the reader to judge the validity of the conclusions and inferences that are drawn in published research.

Four simple questions can be used for identifying the general strength of a study's design (Fig. 3.2). The four questions are considered as follows.

QUESTION 1: WAS AN INTERVENTION APPLIED?

If the investigator actively applies an intervention, the study design is considered to be *experimental*; if he or she does not, the study design is considered to be *observational*.

QUESTION 2: WERE THE SUBJECTS ASSIGNED TO GROUPS?

In an experimental design, if the subjects were randomly assigned to an intervention-versus-control group, the design can be further characterized as being a *true-experimental* study; if the subjects were not, for example the

Table 3.1 Stress-fracture risk factors: possible mechanisms and interrelationships

Risk factor	Mechanisms and interrelationships
Low bone density	Decreased bone strength
Small bone size	Decreased bone strength
Skeletal alignment	Elevated bone strain Unaccustomed bone strain Muscle fatigue
Body size and composition	Elevated bone strain Menstrual disturbances Muscle fatigue Low bone density
Bone turnover	Low bone density Elevated bone strain Inadequate repair of microdamage
Muscle flexibility and joint range	Elevated bone strain Unaccustomed bone strain Muscle fatigue
Muscle strength and endurance	Elevated bone strain Unaccustomed bone strain
Low calcium intake	Greater rate of bone turnover Low bone density Inadequate repair of microdamage
Nutritional factors	Altered body composition Low bone density Greater rate of bone turnover Reduced calcium absorption Menstrual disturbances Inadequate repair of microdamage

Table 3.1 continues.

Table 3.1 *continued*

Risk factor	Mechanisms and interrelationships
Menstrual disturbances	Low bone density Greater rate of bone remodeling Increased calcium excretion
Training	Elevated bone strain Unaccustomed bone strain Greater number of loading cycles Muscle fatigue Inadequate time for repair of microdamage Menstrual disturbances Altered body composition
Inappropriate surface	Elevated bone strain Unaccustomed bone strain Muscle fatigue
Inappropriate footwear	Elevated bone strain Unaccustomed bone strain Muscle fatigue
Higher external loading	Elevated bone strain Muscle fatigue
Genetic factors	Low bone density Greater rate of bone remodeling Psychological traits
Psychological traits	Excessive training Nutritional intake and eating disorders

investigator assigned them to various groups, the design is referred to as a *quasi-experimental* study. If there is no assignment to groups, for example if all the subjects receive the intervention, the design is considered to be *pre-experimental* in nature.

The random-assignment issue is important, because confounding variables are thereby able to be balanced, and some assurance is provided that all the groups are equivalent at the start of the study. Because of this assumption, after the intervention the differences between the groups are able to be attributed to the intervention itself.

One type of true-experimental design that is often used in medical research is the randomized clinical trial. The design's weakness is that random assignment is not always possible. The weakness of quasi-experimental designs is that differences between the groups may be due to existence of bias when the subjects were assigned to groups.

Although this study design provides the strongest evidence for some intervention's preventive or treatment effect, in the clinical setting the design is often impractical, unethical or impossible (for example in study of risk factors such as foot type or bone density).

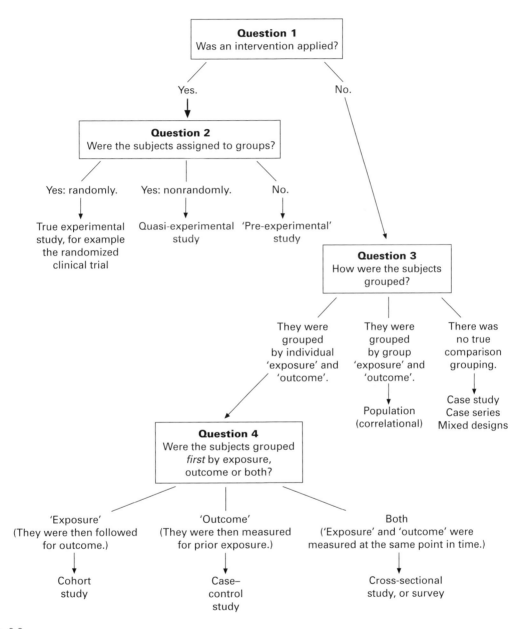

Fig. 3.2
The four questions that can be used for identifying the nature of a study's design.

Experimental studies have been used for researching how calcium supplementation, training-regimen changes, footwear and foot orthoses influence rates of stress-fracture incidence in recruits who are undergoing basic training. To date, no experimental stress-fracture studies have been undertaken among athletes.

QUESTION 3: HOW WERE THE SUBJECTS GROUPED?

In observational designs, the researcher observes the presence or absence of the risk factor and outcome without controlling the factor itself. If true-comparison groups are used, the study design can be considered to be *analytic*; if they are not, it should be considered to be *descriptive*.

Forming true-comparison groups at the outset of the study is important, because the researcher is able to conclude that the differences found between groups are real, not the result of bias or confounding. It is possible that any observed connection or correlation is the result of some as yet unidentified confounder.[2]

If the researcher makes simple comparisons between individuals or a collection of individuals, the study design is referred to as a *case study* or *case series*. Case studies are detailed descriptions of a case of an unusual event or a deadly disease. Case series are descriptions of a number of similar cases or clusters, such as of a type of uncommon stress fracture. If, for example, only one exposure group is studied, without a comparison group, the study is considered to be a *mixed design* (see Chapter 2 about stress-fracture epidemiology).

If the researcher makes simple comparisons between populations, the study design is referred to as being *correlational*. In this type of study, the correlation of two factors in a population is examined. The problem of this design is one of ecological fallacy: the intervention and outcome are not necessarily assessed in the same individuals. The other consideration is that the subjects are grouped according to their individual exposure and outcome, in that case, the ordering of the grouping should be considered.

QUESTION 4: WERE THE SUBJECTS GROUPED FIRST BY EXPOSURE, OUTCOME, OR BOTH?

In the case of observational analytic designs, the researcher passively observes natural events. He or she does this by either assembling a group of exposed and unexposed individuals and following them forward in time in order to examine differences in outcome, or by assembling a stress-fracture group and a control group and studying the two groups for differences in prior exposure to a causal factor.

The former design is referred to as a *cohort*. It is the observational equivalent of an experimental design, because causal inferences are most strongly able to be drawn from it. It is the preferred method for studying rare exposure to or rare causes of injury. The latter design is referred to as *case–control*. It is somewhat easier to conduct and is a good design for studying uncommon stress fractures. Its weakness is that it has more sources of potential error. The various types of observational study are distinguished by the direction of the temporal relationship between observation of the risk factor and stress-fracture occurrence.[3]

PROSPECTIVE COHORT STUDIES

In cohort studies, by way of assembling a group of athletes and measuring the presence of specific risk factors before an injury occurs, the population under study can be monitored longitudinally, or *prospectively*, over a predetermined length of time. The prospective cohort design's greatest strength is that each individual's risk profile is established before the stress fracture has occurred. Its disadvantages are that it is costly and time consuming, because many athletes must be sampled so that enough injuries can be generated in order to support meaningful statistical analysis.[4] Furthermore, there must be some form of accurate (sensitive and specific) injury-surveillance mechanism in order to ensure that stress fractures are detected. Although many large prospective cohort studies have been undertaken in the military, only one study has been reported in athletes.[5]

HISTORICAL COHORT STUDIES

If the investigator uses historical records to identify exposure groups, and those people are contacted to determine the presence or outcome of a stress fracture, the study design is known as *historical cohort*. The weakness of this design is that it is prone to more sources of error (bias and confounding) than a prospective cohort design.

CASE–CONTROL (RETROSPECTIVE) STUDIES

These studies commence with classification of stress-fracture status (is it case or control?), and information about prior exposure to risk factors is obtained. This design is more efficient, because the subjects do not have to be followed over time, and the relative numbers of cases and controls can be closely balanced. However, several problems are associated with it. First, the sample sizes are usually small, which means the subjects are less likely to be representative of the general athlete population. Second, risk-factor documentation is prone to recall bias.

CROSS-SECTIONAL STUDIES, OR SURVEYS

The other, often neglected, possibility is that presence of the risk factor and presence of the outcome (presence or absence of stress fracture) are determined at the same point in time. In these *cross-sectional studies*, or *surveys*, although the appearance may be given that the impact of risk factors can be assessed, cause and effect cannot in fact be established. Unless it can be shown that a (risk) factor preceded injury development, it cannot be assumed that the factor caused the injury.

By strict definition, in a cross-sectional survey, only stress fractures that are present at the time of the survey (injury prevalence) will be recorded. However, in the stress-fracture literature many surveys include injuries from the past, and this may lead to the fact that recall of either risk exposure or injury history is biased. Most studies in the literature about athlete stress fracture are cross-sectional.

Although study design provides a measure of a given study's rigor and thereby a mechanism by which to rank-order a group of studies with reference to the strength of the studies' evidence, factors other than the type of study design impact on the conclusions' validity. Even strong study designs can suffer from having small sample sizes, confounding factors whereby bias is introduced, and problems to do with data analysis and reporting. Also, it is important it be emphasized that in 'weaker' designs, events and phenomena that otherwise would not be 'researchable' are able to be studied.

It is clear that stress-fracture pathogenesis is multifactorial (Table 3.1). In many studies, single risk factors have been investigated among injured and uninjured athletes by way of use of univariate statistical techniques. However, through use of these techniques, interaction of codependent risk factors has tended to be ignored. Multivariate analysis provides a better insight into the relative importance of several risk factors that interact.[6,7]

One of the difficulties involved in evaluating risk factors' role in stress-fracture pathogenesis is that risk factors may be specific to particular stress-fracture sites and to particular athlete populations. For example, a pronated foot may increase the risk for tibial stress fractures whereas a cavus foot may increase the risk for metatarsal stress fractures. Low bone density may play a role in stress fractures in ballet dancers but not in marathon runners. In most studies, the sample sizes are not large enough to enable these risk-factor associations to be analyzed. Grouping together various stress-fracture sites or athlete groups may serve to only mask true relationships between risk factors and stress fractures.

Even if these precautionary considerations are kept in mind, enough studies are reported in the literature to enable a preliminary analysis to be undertaken of the risk factors that are relevant to stress-fracture pathogenesis, and these risk factors warrant more-detailed exploration.

Intrinsic mechanical factors

BONE DENSITY

Low bone density could contribute to development of a stress fracture by way of reduction in bone strength and therefore through increasing the accumulation of microdamage when repetitive loading is undertaken.[8] In the condition osteoporosis, the association between fragility fractures and low bone density is well established, and clinically, bone-density measurements are used in order to predict likelihood of fracture. For example, for age-matched individuals, for every one standard-deviation decrease in bone density at the spine, there is a two-fold increase in risk of spine fracture, and for femoral-neck bone density there is a 2.6-fold increase in hip fracture.[9,10] Before we consider studies in which bone density is examined as being a risk factor for stress fractures in physically active individuals, it is important we review the validity of the techniques that are used for measuring this variable.

MEASUREMENT OF BONE DENSITY

In studies in which the relationship between bone density and stress fractures has been investigated, absorptiometry techniques have been used for measuring bone density. The simplest and oldest of the available quantitative techniques is single photon absorptiometry (SPA), whereby absorbance of low-energy gamma irradiation is measured. However, because it is necessary to have uniform and minimal soft tissue surrounding the bone, only some sites are suitable for scanning. The most popular sites are the distal radius and calcaneus.[11]

To enable other more clinically relevant regions to be measured, dual photon absorptiometry (DPA) was developed, whereby radiation is used at two wavelengths. The technique has now been superseded by dual energy X-ray absorptiometry (DXA), in which the principles are the same as those of DPA but an X-ray tube is used in place of a radio-isotopic source. Compared with DPA, DXA gives improved image resolution, more-stable and more-accurate measurements, lower radiation dose, and reduced scanning time.[12–14] It is now the most widely used clinical and research measure of bone density.

For a DXA scan, the patient lies on a table. The X-ray source (in which alternating pulses are provided at 70 KVP and 140 KVP) is mounted beneath and the X-ray detector above. When the X-ray beam is detected after passing through the patient, it contains information about the patient's characteristics of X-ray absorption. The machine compares this information with the absorption properties of known calibration materials, in order to determine the amount of bone mineral and soft tissue, including fat mass and lean mass. Bone density is calculated by dividing the bone-mineral content (in grams) by the area of bone scanned (bone-mineral density, in grams per centimeter squared). Because DXA measures mass per unit area, literally the term 'bone density' is incorrect. For this reason, many people now refer to DXA density measurements as 'areal density'.

Quantitative computed tomography (QCT) is the only noninvasive method for measuring bone density, whereby a true three-dimensional technique is used as opposed to the areal density of absorptiometric techniques. QCT measurements isolate bone's trabecular component rather than integrate both cortical and trabecular bone in the measurement. Compared with DXA, QCT's disadvantages include lower precision, higher radiation levels, and greater expense; for research purposes, QCT is therefore less acceptable. It has not been used in any of the studies in which bone density has been evaluated as a risk factor for stress fractures.

THE RELATIONSHIP BETWEEN BONE DENSITY AND STRESS-FRACTURE RISK

The results of studies in which the relationship between bone density and stress-fracture risk were investigated are contradictory, as shown in Table 3.2. This may reflect differences in the populations (military or athlete), types of sport (running, dancing, or track and field), measurement techniques (SPA, DPA, or DXA), and bone regions under study.

To date, the relationship between bone density and stress fracture in athlete and military populations has been investigated in seven and four studies, respectively. In most of the athlete studies, women were evaluated (two of the studies included both men and women, four included only women, and one included only men), whereas in most (three out of four) of the military studies, men were evaluated. In three

Table 3.2 *A summary of the studies in which the relationship between bone density and stress fractures was investigated. The studies are ordered according to their study design, then chronologically*

Reference	Study design	Subjects	Sex	Sample size	Technique	Sites	Results: percentage difference (%)†
Giladi et al. 1991[15]	PC	Military	M	91 – SF 198 – NSF	SPA	Tibial shaft	−6.0
Beck et al. 1996[17]	PC	Military	M	23 – SF 587 – NSF	DXA	Femur Tibia Fibula	−3.9* −5.6* −5.2
Bennell et al. 1996[5]	PC	Track and field athletes	F	10 – SF 36 – NSF	DXA	Upper limb Thoracic spine Lumbar spine Femur Tibia and fibula Foot	−3.3 −6.7 −11.9* −2.2 −4.2 −6.6*
			M	10 – SF 39 – NSF	DXA	Upper limb Thoracic spine Lumbar spine Femur Tibia and fibula Foot	−4.9 −4.1 −0.8 −2.9 −4.0 −0.3
Pouilles et al. 1989[18]	XS	Military	M	41 – SF 48 – NSF	DPA	Femoral neck Ward's triangle Trochanter	−5.7* −7.1* −7.4*

Table 3.2 continues.

Table 3.2 continued

Reference	Study design	Subjects	Sex	Sample size	Technique	Sites	Results: percentage difference (%)[†]
Carbon et al. 1990[47]	XS	Various athletes	F	9 – SF 9 – NSF	DPA SPA	Lumbar spine Femoral neck Distal radius Ultradistal radius	–4.0* –7.0 –7.7 0
Frusztajer et al. 1990[86]	CC and XS	Ballet dancers	F	10 – SF 10 – NSF	DPA SPA	Lumbar spine First metatarsal Radial shaft	–4.1 0 0
Myburgh et al. 1990[48]	XS	Various athletes	M and F	25 – SF 25 – NSF (19 F and 6 M)	DXA	Lumbar spine Femoral neck Ward's triangle Trochanter Intertrochanter Proximal femur	–8.5* –6.7* –9.0* –8.6* –5.5 –6.5*
Grimston et al. 1991[19]	XS	Runners	F	6 – SF 8 – NSF	DPA	Lumbar spine Femoral neck Tibial shaft	8.2* 7.6* 9.7
Bennell et al. 1995[88]	XS	Track and field athletes	F	22 – SF 31 – NSF	DXA	Lumbar spine Lower limb Tibia and fibula	–3.5 –0.9 –2.0
Cline et al. 1998[45]	XS	Military	F	49 – SF 78 – NSF	DXA	Lumbar spine Femoral neck Ward's triangle Trochanter Radial shaft	–2.4 0 –2.2 0 1.5
Crossley et al. 1999[16]	XS	Athletes	M	23 – SF 23 – NSF	DXA	Tibial shaft	8.1

*Notes: * = Statistically significant. † Results are given as the percentage difference whereby the stress-fracture subjects (SF) are compared with the non-stress-fracture subjects (NSF). PC = Observational analytic prospective cohort. CC = Case–control. XS = Observational descriptive cross-sectional. DPA = Dual photon absorptiometry. DXA = Dual energy X-ray absorptiometry. SPA = Single photon absorptiometry. F = Females. M = Males.*
(Source: Adapted and reproduced, with permission, from Brukner PD and Bennell KL. Stress Fractures: Critical Reviews in Physical and Rehabilitation Medicine 1997; 9: 151–190, and Bennell et al. Skeletal effects of menstrual disturbances in athletes. Scandinavian Journal of Science and Medicine in Sport 1997; 7: 261–273.)

studies, prospective cohort designs were used and cohort numbers ranged from 95 to 610, whereas in the other studies, cross-sectional designs were used and the stress-fracture group numbers ranged from 6 to 49. With reference to the cross-sectional studies, one problem is that the stress fracture and nonstress fracture groups were often inadequately matched and differed in relation to other factors that are believed to influence bone density and stress-fracture risk, such as menstrual status, body composition, and training level. Multivariate statistical analyses were not undertaken in order to take into account the influence of these confounding factors. It was also unclear how long after the injury the bone-density measurements were taken. It is possible that forced immobilization or a reduced activity level after the stress fracture led to a decrease in bone density.

For osteoporotic fractures, bone-density measurements of the bone at risk of fracture are usually the best predictor of eventual fracture, although measurement of bone density at other sites is also a predictor. Ideally, to provide evidence for a causal relationship between low bone density and stress fracture, measurements are taken at bone sites in which stress fractures occur. In seven studies, bone-density measurements at lower-limb sites were included, whereas in the other studies, only the lumbar spine, radius and/or proximal femur were measured. The latter three sites may not necessarily reflect the bone status at stress-fracture sites.

With reference to men, very little prospective evidence exists in support of a clear causal relationship between bone density and risk of stress fractures. Giladi *et al.*[15] found no difference between the tibial bone density of 91 recruits who developed a stress fracture and 198 recruits who acted as controls. This result held when the data were analyzed for all stress fractures combined, as well as for only femoral and tibial fractures. Similar findings were reported in a cross-sectional study by Crossley *et al.*,[16] who failed to find a difference between the tibial bone density of male runners who had and male runners who did not have a history of tibial stress fracture, as well as by Bennell *et al.*,[5] who used DXA to prospectively assess bone density at a number of regions in male track and field athletes. Although Beck *et al.*[17] found significantly lower tibial and femoral bone density in 23 male recruits who developed a stress fracture compared with 587 controls who did not, the result may be explained by the fact that there were differences in body weight: the stress-

fracture recruits were 11% lighter. Because body weight is a major predictor of bone density, it is important it be ensured that either the groups are matched with reference to this factor or the factor is controlled statistically, otherwise the independent relationship between bone density and stress fractures will not be able to be determined.

In a cross-sectional study, lower bone density was shown at the femoral neck, Ward's triangle, and trochanter in forty-one male recruits who had a stress fracture, compared with twenty-eight male recruits who did not have a stress fracture.[18] None of the other studies among men included these proximal femoral sites, so direct comparisons cannot be made. When the group was subdivided according to fracture site, femoral bone density remained lower in recruits who had a femoral ($n = 12$) or a calcaneal stress fracture ($n = 10$) but not in recruits who had a tibial, fibular or metatarsal fracture ($n = 19$). This site difference may be the result of differences in the proportion of cortical to trabecular bone, and highlights the problem of the measurement site's specificity.

Conversely, in women, some evidence exists that suggests that lower bone density may have a role in stress-fracture development. In the only prospective cohort study to date, female track and field athletes who sustained a stress fracture had significantly lower total-body bone-mineral content and lower bone density at the lumbar spine and foot than female athletes who did not sustain a fracture.[5] The subgroup of women who developed a tibial stress fracture had 8.1% lower bone density at the tibia–fibula. This deficit located at the fracture site supports a possible cause-and-effect relationship, although the number of women in the subgroup was small.

An important point to note is that although bone density was lower in the athletes who had a stress fracture, it remained higher than or similar to the bone density of less active nonathletes. This implies that the level of bone density that physically active people require for short-term bone health may be greater than that required by the general population. It also implies that based on normative DXA values, the stress-fracture individuals in the study would not have been identified as being at risk. At the time of writing, there were no normative databases specific to athletes in various sports, so legitimate comparisons of an individual's bone density cannot be made.

With reference to the cross-sectional studies in female athletes, the findings are contradictory. Again, this may reflect the small sample sizes, as well as differences between the types of sport, the measurement techniques used, and the bone regions assessed. In one study of fourteen female runners, significantly higher lumbar-spine and femoral-neck bone density was actually found in the stress-fracture group.[19] The researchers speculated that greater external loading forces measured in the stress-fracture subjects during running may have been responsible for the runners' higher bone density. This may instead be a spurious result, because of the fact that there were only six athletes in the stress-fracture group and eight athletes in the control group. In other studies, either no difference or significantly lower bone density has been reported in the stress-fracture group.

The relationship between bone density and stress-fracture development remains not clearly established, although evidence exists that the risk factor of low bone density may be more common in women. Conflicting results from studies could indicate that the population of athletes who have a stress fracture is heterogeneous in relation to bone density, and that other factors that are independent of bone mass contribute to risk of fracture, particularly in men. It would seem that bone densitometry generally does not have a place as a screening tool for predicting risk of stress fracture in otherwise healthy individuals. However, bone densitometry may be warranted in athletes who have multiple stress-fracture episodes and in females who have menstrual disturbance.

BONE GEOMETRY

Bone strength is related to not only bone-mineral density but bone geometry. For bones loaded in tension or compression, the amount of load the bone can withstand before failing is proportional to the bone's cross-sectional area. The larger the area, the stronger and stiffer the bone. For bending and torsional loads, both the cross-sectional area and the cross-sectional moments of inertia will determine bone strength. Bones that have a larger cross-sectional area and in which bone tissue is distributed further away from the neutral axis will be stronger when subjected to load and will therefore be less likely to fracture.[20]

The structural properties of long bones vary with age and gender, and are mostly dependent on body size.[21] However, variation in bone geometry is great even between individuals of similar age and build; there is, in fact, much greater variation in structural geometry than between bone-material properties, including bone-mineral density.[22] Differences in bone geometry might therefore partly explain differences in stress-fracture predisposition.

In a prospective observational cohort study of 295 male Israeli military recruits, it was found that the recruits who developed a stress fracture had narrower tibias in the mediolateral plane at three levels (measured by using radiographs), compared with the recruits who did not have a stress fracture.[23] This result was found for total stress fractures as well as for stress fractures only in the tibia and only in the femur. The researchers suggested that the reason the result was seen for femoral stress fractures as well was that the size of the tibia is an indication of the size of tubular bones in general.

In further work by the same research group, these widths were used in order to calculate the cross-sectional moment of inertia. Using multivariate statistical techniques, the group found that for stress-fracture risk, the cross-sectional moment of inertia about the anteroposterior axis (CSMIAP), an estimate of bone's ability to resist bending, was an even better indicator than tibial width.[24] Thirty-one percent of recruits who had a low CSMIAP developed a tibial stress fracture, compared with only 14% of recruits who had a high CSMIAP.[25] However, it must be pointed out that tibial geometry is complex, and that it changes continuously along the length of the tibia. The researchers derived tibial widths from standard radiographs, and based their calculations on the assumption that the tibia is an elliptical ring that has an eccentric hole. However, their assumption may not be valid. From our experience, tibial cross-sectional shape varies widely between individuals, and in many cases is closer to a triangle than to an ellipse.

Nevertheless, the results in which differences in tibial geometry were revealed between recruits who had a stress fracture and recruits who did not have a stress fracture were supported by a recent prospective study of more than 600 military recruits who were undergoing 12 weeks of basic training. Bone-mineral data acquired from a DXA scanner were used to derive cross-sectional geometric properties of the tibia, fibula, and femur.[17] This method is likely to be more accurate than radiographs, because it does not entail making assumptions about cross-sectional shape and manual measurements of cortical thickness.

The results showed that compared with the recruits who did not have a stress fracture, even after adjusting for differences in body weight, the recruits who had a stress fracture had a smaller tibial width ($P = 0.03$), a smaller cross-sectional area ($P = 0.03$), a smaller moment of inertia ($P = 0.07$), and a smaller modulus ($P = 0.05$); in fact, the stress-fracture subjects' average reduction in tibial bone geometry seems to be similar to the results from the Israeli study (Fig. 3.3).

Another interesting finding in the study by Beck and colleagues is that in the fracture group, the smaller dimensions were limited to long-bone diaphyses, not joint size, which suggests a specificity in the structural deficit in the fracture group. Evidence exists that compared with joint size, diaphyseal cross-sectional dimensions are more environmentally influenced. This could indicate that the stress fracture group's bones

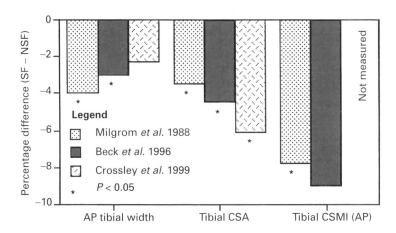

Fig. 3.3
The average percentage difference between the stress-fracture (SF) group and the non-stress-fracture group (NSF) for tibial-geometry measurements in the studies by Milgrom *et al.*,[24] Beck *et al.*[17] and Crossley *et al.*[16] *Note:* AP, CSA and CSMI stand for antero-posterior, cross-sectional area, and cross-sectional moment of inertia, respectively. Percentage difference = (SF − NSF)/NSF × 100. The values for Beck *et al.*[17] are adjusted for differences in body weight. The values for Milgrom *et al.*[24] are non-weight adjusted, and are the mean of measurements at two locations in the distal half of the tibia.

had not been sufficiently loaded before basic training in order to develop cortices strong enough to withstand the subsequent stresses.

In military recruits who are subjected to intense, unaccustomed physical activity, the presence of smaller and weaker bones may lead to a higher rate of bone microdamage. If there is inadequate time for adaptive cortical remodeling to occur, a stress fracture could result. Evidence also exists that suggests that having a smaller bone is a risk factor for stress fractures in athletes, even though the athletes' bones are loaded more gradually over a longer period of time. In a cross-sectional study of forty-six male runners, CT scanning was used to evaluate tibial geometry at the level of the middle and distal third.[16] Compared with the runners who did not have a stress fracture, the runners who had a history of tibial stress fracture had a significantly smaller tibial cross-sectional area (after adjustments had been made for body mass and height) (Fig. 3.3). Whether or not this is also a risk factor in female athletes has yet to be investigated.

Even if bone geometry has a role in stress-fracture development, its clinical relevance as a risk factor is limited. Large-scale screening of tibial geometry in which plain radiographs or DXA techniques are used is impractical and costly. Further research might make it possible to develop surrogate indicators of tibial geometry via simple anthropometric measurements.

SKELETAL ALIGNMENT

Lower-limb and foot alignment may predispose a person to stress fractures through either creation of stress-concentration areas in bone or promotion of muscle fatigue. Although in military populations an association has been sought between various factors that influence skeletal alignment and stress fracture, few data exist that pertain to athletes. Furthermore, the ways in which the factors were defined and measured are inconsistent, and the measure-

ments' reliability and validity were often not addressed. The studies in which the link between skeletal alignment and stress fractures has been attempted to be evaluated are summarized in Table 3.3.

The foot's structure will help determine how much force is absorbed by the foot and how much force is transferred to bone during ground contact. The high-arched (pes cavus) foot is more rigid and less able to absorb shock, so more force passes to the tibia and femur. The low-arched (pes planus) foot is more flexible, as stress is able to be absorbed by the foot's musculoskeletal structures. The low-arched foot is also less stable during weightbearing, and this may contribute to muscle fatigue, because the muscles have to work harder in order to control the excessive motion, especially at toe-off.

Theoretically, either foot type could predispose a person to a stress fracture. Several studies have indicated that the risk of stress fracture is greater for male recruits who have a high foot arch than for male recruits who have a low foot arch.[26–28] In a prospective cohort study, the overall incidence of stress fracture in the low-arched (pes planus) group was 10%, as opposed to 40% in the high-arched group.[26] A similar trend was noted when tibial and femoral stress fractures were analyzed separately. However, assessment of foot type was based on observation of the feet when they were in a nonfunctional position, and the recruits who had extreme pes planus were excluded. Furthermore, the trainees who had an 'average' arch had a stress-fracture incidence – 31% – similar to that of the high-arched trainees.

Nevertheless, these findings were supported in a cross-sectional study in which a contact-pressure display method was used to provide foot–ground pressure patterns and derived stress-intensity parameters.[28] In the study, recruits who had a high arch were more likely to have sustained a stress fracture than were recruits who had a lower arch. By contrast, an association between foot type and stress-fracture

Table 3.3 *The studies in which the association between skeletal alignment and stress fractures has been investigated. Studies are ranked first according to their study design, and second according to chronology*

Reference	Study design	Subjects	Sample size	Factors analyzed	Measurement method	Results
Friberg 1982[36]	XS and PC	Army – Finland	371 – M	Leg-length difference	X-ray – WB	Increased incidence with increased difference
Giladi *et al.* 1985[26]	PC	Army – Israel	295 – M	Foot type	Observation – NWB	SF risk greater in high arch than in low arch
Giladi *et al.* 1987[50]	PC	Army – Israel	295 – M	Genu valgum and varum	Observation	No relationship to SF
				Tibial torsion	NS	No relationship to SF
				Gait in-toe and out-toe	Observation	No relationship to SF
Montgomery *et al.* 1989[29]	PC	SEAL – United States	505 – M	Genu recurvatum	Distance heels to bed – supine	No relationship to SF
				Genu valgum and varum	Distance between condyles – WB	No relationship to SF
				Q angle	Goniometer – supine	No relationship to SF
				Foot type	Observation – WB	No relationship to SF
Simkin *et al.* 1989[27]	PC	Army – Israel	295 – M	Foot type	X-ray – WB	High arch – higher risk of femoral and tibial SF
						Low arch – higher risk of MT SF
Milgrom *et al.* 1994[51]	PC	Army – Israel	783 – M	Genu valgum and varum	Distance between condyles	No relationship to SF
Bennell *et al.* 1996[5]	PC	Athletes	53 – F and 58 – M	Leg-length difference	Tape measure – NWB	Leg-length difference – higher risk of SF
				Genu valgum and varum	Observation – NWB	No relationship to SF
				Foot type	Observation – WB	No relationship to SF
Cowan *et al.* 1996[35]	PC	Army – United States	294 – M	Genu valgum and varum	Computer digitization of photographs, showing highlighted anatomic landmarks – WB	Increased SF risk with increased valgus
				Genu recurvatum		No relationship to SF
				Q angle		Q angle >15° = increased risk for SF
				Leg-length difference		No relationship to SF
Winfield *et al.* 1997[38]	PC	Marines – United States	101 – F	Q angle	NS	No relationship to SF
Hughes 1985[52]	XS	Army – United States	47 – M	Forefoot varus	Goniometer – NWB	Greater FFV 8.3 times at risk of MT SF
				Rearfoot valgus	Goniometer – WB	No relationship to SF

Table 3.3 continues.

Table 3.3 continued

Reference	Study design	Subjects	Sample size	Factors analysed	Measurement method	Results
Brunet et al. 1990[37]	XS	Athletes	375 – F and 1130 – M	Leg-length difference	Self-report questionnaire	Leg-length difference – higher risk of SF
				Foot type	Self-report questionnaire	No relationship to SF
Brosh and Arcan 1994[28]	XS	NS	42 – M	Foot type	Contact-pressure display	Higher arches = increased risk of SF
Ekenman et al. 1996[33]	XS	Athletes	29 – SF M and F	Foot type	Contact pressure during gait	No relationship to SF
			30 – NSF M and F	Rearfoot valgus	NS	No relationship to SF
				Forefoot varus	NS	No relationship to SF
Matheson et al. 1987[32]	CS	Athletes	320	Subtalar varus	NS	Not related to SF site
				Foot type	NS	Pronated – tibial and tarsal SF; cavus – MT and femoral SF
				Forefoot varus	NS	Not related to SF site
				Genu valgum and varum	Distance between condyles	Not related to SF site
				Tibial varum	NS	Not related to SF site

Notes: CS = Case series. PC = Prospective cohort. XS = Cross-sectional. M = Male. F = Female. NS = Not stated. NWB = Non-weightbearing. WB = Weightbearing. MT = Metatarsal. SF = Stress fracture. NSF = Non-stress fracture. FFV = Forefoot varus.

risk has not been reported in all military studies. Montgomery and colleagues[29] used visual inspection of foot posture during standing, and found that the incidence of stress fracture was similar in recruits who had cavus, neutral, or planus feet. However, a relationship between foot type and stress fracture may vary, depending on the stress-fracture site. When radiographs were used to assess foot type, femoral and tibial stress fractures were more prevalent when higher arches were present, whereas incidence of metatarsal fractures was higher when lower arches were present.[27] Therefore, researchers may fail to find an association between specific foot types and stress fractures, because they have not grouped the data according to stress-fracture site.

Most of the studies in athletes are case series in which a comparison of injured and uninjured

athletes is unable to be made. Although pes planus may be the most common foot type among stress-fracture athletes who present to sports clinics,[30,31] pes planus may be equally as common among athletes who remain uninjured. In a large series of 320 stress fractures, pes planus was more frequent in athletes who had a tibial or a tarsal bone stress fracture and was least common in athletes who had a metatarsal stress fracture.[32] This finding tends to differ from military findings, which are that foot fractures seem to be more prevalent in recruits who have pes planus.

In the only prospective cohort study in athletes, foot type that was assessed visually during weightbearing was not a predictor of the likelihood of stress fracture.[5] However, the numbers were insufficient for evaluating the results according to stress-fracture site. Even when a single stress-fracture site was being assessed, foot type measured by way of contact pressure from a force platform during walking did not seem to have a role. In twenty-nine consecutive patients who presented with a unilateral tibial stress fracture, there was no difference in foot type between injured and uninjured legs or between injured athletes and a reference group of thirty sedentary and athletic individuals.[33]

A leg-length discrepancy has been postulated as being a potential risk factor for stress fracture, because of resulting skeletal realignment and asymmetries in loading, bone torsion, and muscle contraction.[34] In one study in male recruits, no relationship was found between leg-length differences (measured from photographs by way of computer digitization of highlighted landmarks) and likelihood of stress fractures.[35]

However, the results of all other studies in this area do suggest an association. Using a radiologic method to assess leg length during standing, Friberg[36] found that in 130 cases of stress fracture in military recruits, the longer leg was associated with 73% of tibial, metatarsal, and femoral fractures, whereas 60% of fibular fractures were found in the shorter leg. In a prospective analysis whereby a group of 102 parachutists were followed over 330 days, Friberg observed there was a positive correlation between the extent of leg-length inequality and stress-fracture incidence. Incidence of stress fractures in people who had equal leg length was 15.4%. This increased to 24.3% in people who had between 5 and 9 millimeters' difference and to 66.7% in people who had between 15 and 20 millimeters' difference. However, no statistical analyses were undertaken to assess the significance of the results.

Similar findings have been reported in a cross-sectional survey of male and female runners. Using a self-administered questionnaire, the runners who claimed to have a leg-length difference were more likely to have sustained a stress fracture in the past.[37] In a cohort study, 70% of the women who developed a stress fracture had a leg-length difference of more than 0.5 centimeters (measured by using a tape measure in supine), compared with 36% of women who did not have a stress fracture.[5] Based on these reports, it would seem to be appropriate that leg-length discrepancies be corrected should they exist.

The other alignment features that have been assessed in relation to stress fractures include the presence of genu varum, genu valgum, or genu recurvatum, an increased Q angle, and tibial torsion. Of these, only the Q angle has been found in association with stress fractures. In a study in which computer digitization of highlighted landmarks from photographs was used, male recruits who had a Q angle of more than 15° had a relative risk of stress fracture that was 5.4 times that of recruits who had an angle of less than 15°.[35] Conversely, in other studies, no relationship has been found between Q angle and stress-fracture occurrence.[29,38]

Although the literature suggests that foot type may have a role in stress-fracture development, the exact relationship may depend on the injured region's anatomic location and the activities undertaken by the person. However, a leg-length discrepancy does seem to be a risk factor in both military and civilian populations. The failure to find an association between other biomechanical features and stress fractures in cohort studies does not necessarily rule out the importance of these features for individuals. A thorough biomechanic assessment is an essential part of both treatment and prevention of stress fractures. Until biomechanic abnormalities' contribution to stress-fracture risk is clarified through scientific research, correction of the abnormalities should be attempted, if possible. This is particularly the case for people who present with a recurrent stress fracture.

BODY SIZE AND COMPOSITION

Theoretically, body size and soft-tissue composition could affect stress-fracture risk directly, by influencing the forces applied to bones. For example, because body weight is positively related to ground-reaction force, heavier individuals would generate higher forces during physical activity,[39] and the likelihood of stress fracture could thereby increase. Body size and composition could also have indirect effects on stress-fracture risk by influencing bone density or menstrual function. Smaller, leaner athletes are more likely to have lower bone density, because body weight, lean mass, and fat mass are all significant determinants of bone density. Similarly, menstrual disturbances are more prevalent among female athletes who are light and do not have much body fat.

A number of potential risk factors related to body size and composition have been reported in the stress-fracture literature, including height, weight, body-mass index (BMI), skinfold thickness, total and regional lean mass and fat mass, limb and segment lengths, and body girths and widths. Measurements have usually been obtained by way of simple anthropometric techniques, although in one study, DXA was used to measure fat and lean mass.[5]

Although the role of body-habitus variables has been evaluated in several studies, no researchers have reported differences in height, weight, body-mass index or fat mass for athletes who have sustained a stress fracture, compared with athletes who have not.[5,40–43] Failure to find an association between these factors and stress-fracture incidence may be because of the fact that athletes who play a specific sport tend to be relatively homogeneous in terms of somatotype and body composition. Also, any relationship that exists may be nonlinear. For example, although both lighter and heavier athletes may be at risk, the data have not been analyzed appropriately in order to detect this relationship. Furthermore, these parameters are unlikely to be

stable, and their measurement in cross-sectional studies may not reflect their status before the injury occurred.

Body size may be a risk factor among military recruits, the size variations of whom are likely to be greater than those of athletes. In a recent study, stress-fracture incidence was greater among smaller individuals.[17] The researchers surmised that this was because of common training requirements, whereby similar weight packs and other equipment were carried regardless of the recruits' body weight. It is also possible that the fracture group's lower body-mass index was indicative of relatively lower muscle mass and/or poorer physical conditioning before training commenced. On the other hand, overweight individuals may be at increased risk of stress fracture, because they also tend to be less physically active. However, in many military studies, among both men and women an association between stress fractures and various parameters of body size and composition has failed to be found.[15,38,44,45]

In female Marine trainees, a narrow pelvis (≤ 26 centimeters) was associated with a greater risk of stress fracture ($P < 0.09$).[38] Stress-fracture incidence in the women who had a narrow pelvis was 14%, compared with 4% in the women who had a wider pelvis. The relative risk of stress fracture was therefore 3.57 for recruits who had a narrow pelvis compared with 'normals'. An explanation for this finding is not clear, because a wider pelvis has typically been attributed to increased biomechanic stresses through an increase in the Q angle. It is possible that a narrow pelvis in this group of female Marines is a marker for some other risk factor for stress fractures.

In general, no consistent relationships have been observed between body size or composition and stress-fracture risk. However, monitoring body fat and lean mass may be useful for indicating health and nutritional status, particularly in female athletes, among whom disordered patterns of eating are relatively common.

Physiological factors

BONE TURNOVER

It is evident that bone remodeling has a role in stress-fracture pathogenesis, and that perturbations in bone remodeling, either generalized or focal, may predispose a person to stress fracture. Stress fractures develop if microdamage cannot be successfully repaired through the remodeling process, and they therefore accumulate to form symptomatic 'macrocracks' in bone. However, accelerated remodeling, which results from either excessive bone strain or the influence of systemic factors, may also weaken bone, because bone resorption occurs before new bone is formed. This could enable microdamage to accumulate, and repetitive mechanical loading to occur at remodeling sites. Conversely, depressed bone remodeling, in particular bone formation, may not enable normal skeletal repair of naturally occurring microdamage to occur. It is conceivable that either sequence could lead to development of a stress fracture in individuals who are training intensively.

In humans, because direct assessment of bone remodeling is invasive and impractical, measurement of biochemical markers of bone turnover may prove to be useful in a clinical setting, in order to aid identification of people who are most at risk for stress fracture. In a prospective cohort study of 104 male military recruits, it was found that a single measurement of plasma hydroxyproline (a nonspecific indicator of bone resorption), which was taken during the first week of a training program, was significantly higher in five recruits who subsequently sustained a stress fracture than in the recruits who remained uninjured.[46] Although this finding supports the concept that elevated bone turnover may be a stimulus for stress-fracture development, hydroxyproline is not specific to bone, and the elevated levels therefore may well reflect nonskeletal sources.

In a limited number of cross-sectional studies, biochemical markers of bone turnover have been measured among small samples of female athletes who have and do not have a history of stress fracture.[41,47,48] In these studies, no difference has been found in bone-turnover levels between groups; however, single measurements of less sensitive markers were taken at variable times after diagnosis was undertaken.

In a twelve-month prospective study, bone turnover was evaluated in forty-six female and forty-nine male track and field athletes who were seventeen to twenty-six years of age and of whom twenty developed a stress fracture.[49] Baseline levels of bone turnover were evaluated in all athletes, and monthly bone-turnover levels were evaluated in a subset that consisted of the twenty athletes who sustained a stress fracture and a matched comparison group the members of which did not sustain a stress fracture. Bone formation was assessed by using serum osteocalcin, and bone resorption by urinary excretion of pyridinium cross-links and N-telopeptides of Type I collagen. The athletes who developed a stress fracture had a similar baseline level of bone turnover compared with their counterparts who did not have a stress fracture, and serial measurements revealed no differences in average levels of bone turnover between the athletes who developed a stress fracture and the control group. Also, in the athletes who had a stress fracture, no difference was recorded in bone-turnover levels either before or following the onset of bony pain (Fig. 3.4).

These results show that for athletes, single and multiple measurements of bone turnover are not clinically useful predictors of the likelihood of stress fractures. However, they do not negate the possibility of the pathogenetic role of local changes in bone remodeling at stress-fracture sites, given the high biologic variability of bone-turnover markers, and the fact that bone-turnover levels reflect the integration of all bone remodeling throughout the skeleton. If trabecular bone, which has greater metabolic activity,

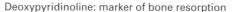

Deoxypyridinoline: marker of bone resorption

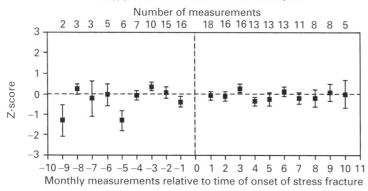

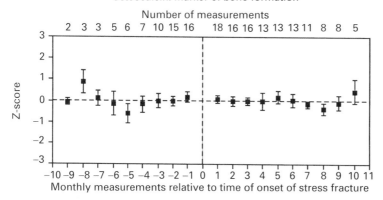

Fig. 3.4

The median z-score (SE) for each monthly bone-turnover measurement among athletes who had a stress fracture. The number of measurements at each time point is shown across the top of each graph. The zero month represents the first onset of stress-fracture pain. The negative months are the ones preceding the stress fracture, and the positive months are the ones following the stress fracture. (Source: Adapted and reproduced, with permission, from Bennell *et al.* A 12-month prospective study of the relationship between stress fractures and bone turnover in athletes. *Calcified Tissue International* 1998; 63: 80–85.)

contributes to bone-turnover levels more than cortical bone does, this may explain why bone-turnover markers are relatively insensitive to stress fractures, which are mainly cortical lesions.

MUSCLE FLEXIBILITY, AND JOINT RANGE OF MOTION

Flexibility of muscles and joints may directly influence stress-fracture risk by way of altering the forces applied to bone. Numerous variables have been assessed, including range of rearfoot inversion–eversion, ankle dorsiflexion–plantarflexion, knee flexion–extension, and hip rotation–extension, together with length of calf, hamstring, quadriceps, hip adductors and hip

flexor muscles (Table 3.4). Of the variables, only range of hip external rotation[15,50,51] and range of ankle dorsiflexion[52] have been associated with stress-fracture development, and even these findings have been inconsistent.

In the Israeli military, large prospective cohort studies included an orthopedic examination as well as assessment of other risk factors for stress fracture.[15,51] The soldiers in whom hip external rotation was greater than 65° had risk for tibial and total stress fractures that was higher than that of the soldiers whose range was less than 65°. The risk for tibial stress fracture increased 2% for every 1° increase in hip external-rotation range.[51] However, in two prospective studies, one in male American recruits[29] and the other in male and female athletes,[5] these findings failed

Table 3.4 *The studies in which the association between muscle and joint flexibility and stress fractures has been investigated. The studies are ranked first according to the strength of their study design, and second according to chronology*

Reference	Study design	Subjects	Sample size	Factors analyzed	Measurement method	Results
Giladi et al. 1987[50]	PC	Army – Israel	295 – M	Hip Int and Ext rotation	Goniometer – hip 90° Fl	Increased risk of SF with greater Ext rotation
				Ankle DF and PF	Goniometer – knee 90° Fl	No relationship to SF
				Rearfoot Inv and Ev	Goniometer	No relationship to SF
				Generalized lig laxity	Thumb-extension test	No relationship to SF
Montgomery et al. 1989[29]	PC	SEAL – United States	505 – M	Hip E	Thomas test – distance to table	No relationship to SF
				Hip Int and Ext rotation	Goniometer – prone	No relationship to SF
				Knee Ext and Flex	Passive – distance	No relationship to SF
				Ankle DF	Knee ext – distance	No relationship to SF
Milgrom et al. 1994[51]	PC	Army – Israel	783 – M	Hip Ext rotation	Goniometer – hip 90° Fl	Increased risk of SF with greater Ext rotation
Bennell et al. 1996[5]	PC	Athletes	53 – F and 58 – M	Hamstring and LSp	Sit-and-reach test	No relationship to SF
				Hip Int and Ext rotation	Goniometer – hip 90° Fl and E	No relationship to SF
				Ankle DF	DF lunge test – distance	No relationship to SF
				Calf length	Goniometer – knee ext	No relationship to SF
Winfield et al. 1997[38]	PC	Marines – United States	101 – F	Rearfoot Inv and Ev	Goniometer – passive	No relationship to SF
Hughes 1985[52]	XS	Army – United States	47 – M	Ankle DF	Goniometer – NWB passive	Reduced range 4.6 times at risk of MT SF
Ekenman et al. 1996[33]	XS	Athletes	29 – SF M and F	Big toe Fl and E	NS	No relationship to SF
			30 – NSF M and F	Ankle DF and PF	NS	No relationship to SF
				Rearfoot Inv and Ev	NS	No relationship to SF
				Hamstrings	NS	No relationship to SF
				Quadriceps	NS	No relationship to SF
				Hip adductors	NS	No relationship to SF
				Hip flexors	NS	No relationship to SF

Notes: PC = Prospective cohort. XS = Cross-sectional. M = Male. F = Female. NSF = Non-stress fracture. NS = Not stated. MT = Metatarsal. SF = Stress fracture. DF = Dorsiflexion. Int = Internal. Ext = External. LSp = Lumbar spine. Inv = Inversion. Ev = Eversion. Fl = Flexion. E = Extension. DF = Dorsiflexion. PF = Plantarflexion.

to be confirmed. It is possible that the Israeli recruits represent a separate population, because their average hip external-rotation range was much higher than that reported for other populations.

In a cross-sectional study of forty-seven male recruits, restricted ankle-joint dorsiflexion was related to an increased risk of metatarsal stress fracture.[52] The recruits who had a reduced range were 4.6 times more likely to develop a metatarsal stress fracture. Conversely, other researchers have measured ankle dorsiflexion and have failed to find a relationship. This may be because the data were analyzed for all stress-fracture sites combined, and this may have masked a true relationship.

The difficulty involved in assessing the role of muscle and joint flexibility in stress fractures may be related to a number of factors, including the relatively imprecise measurement methods, the heterogeneity of these variables, and the fact that both increased and decreased flexibility may contribute. From a clinical perspective, assessment of muscle and joint flexibility should be included in prevention and management of stress fractures until scientific evidence leads to clarification of the role of these factors. If individuals are found to have restricted flexibility in comparison with individuals who are of a similar age and who play a similar sport, measures can be introduced for stretching the tight structures. If increased flexibility is noted, it is important it be ensured that there is adequate muscular stabilization in order to control the greater range of motion.

MUSCULAR STRENGTH AND ENDURANCE

Skeletal muscle may play a dual role in stress-fracture development. Some researchers consider that muscles act dynamically and that stress fractures are thereby caused by an increase in bone strain at sites of muscle attachment.[53,54] If this is the injury mechanism for stress fractures, larger and stronger muscles that have greater ability to generate force should be associated with an increased risk for stress fracture. Although there are no experimental studies that show that stress fractures develop from muscular pull at bony attachments, this would seem to be true in upper-extremity stress fractures such as those of the ulna or radius among swimmers.

Skeletal muscle attenuates and dissipates forces applied to bone.[55] During running, each foot strikes the ground approximately 500 times per kilometer. Each heel strike generates vertical ground-reaction forces (GRFs) that vary from two to five times body weight.[56,57] The forces can be considerably higher: up to twelve times body weight, during jumping and landing activities.[58] A shock wave traveling in bone results in vibrations from 25 to 100 Hertz.[59] These shock waves travel up the axial skeleton and are attenuated by muscles, bones, and joint structures along the way. For example, 54% of the shock measured at the medial femoral condyle has been absorbed by the time it reaches the forehead.[55] It is therefore evident that bone actually 'sees' only a small fraction of the total force, mostly because of attenuation by muscles.

Muscle weakness or fatigue could therefore predispose a person to stress fracture by causing an increase or a redistribution of stress to bone.[60,61] In military recruits, accelerometry was used to assess the amount of shock transmitted to bone.[62] Vertical accelerations in recruits' tibiae during walking were measured before and after a 24 kilometer fast-cadence march. A control group of soldiers who did not participate in the march was also measured. After the march, there were increases in acceleration amplitudes of between 20% and 30%, which implies that reduced shock-absorption capabilities resulted from skeletal-muscle fatigue.

Using a biomechanic model, Scott and Winter[63] calculated that during running, the tibia is subjected to a large forward bending moment as a result of ground-reaction force. The calf muscles oppose this large bending moment by applying a backward moment as they contract to control the tibia's rotation and the foot's lowering to the ground. The total effect is a smaller bending moment. If we extrapolate from this, a stress fracture could result if the calf muscles are unable to produce adequate eccentric force to counteract the loading at ground contact and to decrease excessive bone strain.

Although muscle strength and muscle fatigue have not been found to be related to stress-fracture occurrence in studies in which they were directly evaluated,[15,33,51] this may be because of the study design or the methods used to assess muscle function. In male recruits, relatively crude tests were used, including isometric quadriceps strength measured at one knee angle, and the number of leg thrusts performed in thirty seconds. Although the measurements were performed just before basic training was undertaken, the methods may not have been sensitive enough to detect differences in muscle strength or endurance between people who had and did not have a stress fracture. In athletes, an isokinetic dynamometer was used to measure maximal concentric strength and endurance (during 100 repetitive maximal concentric contractions) of the ankle plantar-flexor muscles.[33] Unfortunately, the study was cross-sectional in design, so it is impossible to know whether or not the measurements reflect muscle function before the stress fracture occurred. Furthermore, because the calf muscles act eccentrically to reduce bone load at ground contact, it may have been better to evaluate eccentric instead of concentric activity.

There is some indirect evidence that muscle fatigue is a risk factor in stress-fracture development, in a study by Grimston and colleagues.[64] The researchers found that during the later stages of a 45 minute run, women who had a history of stress fracture recorded increased ground-reaction forces, whereas in the control group, ground-reaction forces did not vary during the run. The researchers surmised that this may indicate differences in fatigue adaptation and muscle activity. Although it is probable that muscular fatigue and reduced shock absorption are risk factors for athletes engaged in long-distance running and for recruits involved in extreme physical activity, more research has to be undertaken in order to confirm this contention.

Measurements of muscle size can be indicative of that muscle's ability to generate force. Male recruits who had a larger calf circumference developed significantly fewer femoral and tibial stress fractures.[62] This finding was also evident in female athletes (but not male athletes), whereby every one centimeter decrease in calf girth was associated with a four-fold greater risk of stress fracture.[5] In both studies, the calf girth was corrected for skinfold thickness in order to ensure that the measurement was a better indicator of calf-muscle size. In the military study, the variable of calf-girth circumference was also found to be independent of tibial-bone width. The finding that there was a smaller calf girth in people who went on to develop a stress fracture tends to support the hypothesis that muscles act to protect against rather than cause stress fractures. So that a causal relationship can be established, the effectiveness of a calf-strengthening program in reducing stress-fracture incidence should be evaluated in a randomized, controlled trial.

Hormonal factors

SEX HORMONES

Compared with the general female population, athletes have a higher prevalence of menstrual disturbances, including delayed menarche, anovulation, an abnormal luteal phase, oligomenorrhea, and amenorrhea.[65–67] Younger, nulliparous women who are excessively lean and who train intensely seem to be especially at risk of developing menstrual disturbances. In a questionnaire survey of 226 elite athletes, menstrual disturbances were most prevalent in ballet (52%), gymnastics (100%), lightweight rowing (67%), and distance running (65%), compared with swimming (31%), and team sports (17%).[68] It is therefore evident that menstrual disturbances are relatively common in the female-athlete population.

Stress fractures may, in fact, be more frequent among female athletes who have a menstrual disturbance. The cause may be a lowered estrogen level that results in lower bone density, accelerated bone remodeling or negative calcium balance, or interaction of these variables. Studies have revealed that axial bone density among athletes who have amenorrhea or oligomenorrhea is low compared with that of the athletes' eumenorrheic counterparts and/or sedentary controls.[69–72] Appendicular bone density may also be lower among female athletes who have a menstrual disturbance,[71,72] although this has been a less consistent finding.

Estrogen deficiency generally leads to accelerated bone remodeling. Because bone resorption occurs before bone formation in this process, the bone is in a weakened state and is therefore more likely to accumulate microdamage if subjected to repeated loading. Estrogen loss also causes increased calcium excretion, which can result in negative calcium balance if dietary calcium is inadequate. This may seem analogous to the situation of increased risk of osteoporotic fracture in hypoestrogenic postmenopausal women; however, athletes, in contrast to postmenopausal women, typically sustain their bony injuries in cortical rather than trabecular bone. Furthermore, there may in fact be decreased rather than increased remodeling in women who have athletic amenorrhea.

THE RELATIONSHIP BETWEEN A SHORTENED LUTEAL PHASE AND STRESS FRACTURES

Although amenorrhea is the most obvious sign of reproductive-hormone disturbance, subtle changes in reproductive-hormone levels caused by exercise may be too small to produce amenorrhea. A decrease in progesterone production that is associated with short luteal phases and anovulation can be present in women despite normal menstrual-cycle duration and normal flow characteristics.[73,74] A lowered progesterone level may be detrimental to bone health, because progesterone might promote bone formation, particularly in cortical bone.[75–77] In a prospective study in which eumenorrheic women were involved and in which two-thirds of the women engaged in running, Prior *et al.*[78] found that recurrent short luteal-phase cycles and anovulation are associated with spinal-bone loss of approximately 2% to 4% per year.

Serum-progesterone levels and the proportion of the total menstrual cycle spent in the luteal phase have also been found to be a significant predictor of both lumbar-spine bone density,[79] and rate of change of bone mass at this site.[78] However, in a cross-sectional study, the researchers failed to find a significant difference in spinal-bone density between group members who had a short luteal phase length and group members who had a long luteal phase length.[80] Despite the fact that luteal-phase deficiency could have detrimental effects on bone, a link between the deficiency and stress-fracture risk has yet to be sought.

THE RELATIONSHIP BETWEEN AMENORRHEA, OLIGOMENORRHEA AND STRESS FRACTURES

The relationship between amenorrhea or oligomenorrhea and stress-fracture risk has been the subject of a number of studies, which have mainly been retrospective cross-sectional surveys of runners and ballet dancers.[40–43,81,82] Many of the studies are characterized by small samples and a low questionnaire-response rate. In other studies, the subjects were specifically recruited according to set criteria: either stress-fracture history or menstrual status.[19,47,48,70,83–87] Categorization of menstrual status is based on the number of menses per year rather than on analysis of hormone levels, and definitions of menstrual status vary between studies. When hormonal assessment is included, most measurements are single ones, and are often nonstandardized with reference to the menstrual-cycle phase. Length of exposure to amenorrhea also differs within and between studies, and this may influence stress-fracture risk.

Despite the methodology limitations, the findings generally suggest that stress fractures are more common among athletes who have a menstrual disturbance[5,19,38,40–43,47,48,81,83,84,86,88] (Fig. 3.5 a and b). Athletes who have a menstrual disturbance have a relative risk for stress fracture that is between two and four times greater than that of their eumenorrheic counterparts. However, with reference to ballet dancers, logistic regression analysis revealed that amenorrhea for longer than six months was an independent contributor to stress-fracture risk, and that the estimated risk was ninety-three times that of a dancer who had regular menses.[43] Although this risk seems to be extraordinarily high, the sample of fifty-four dancers included only six dancers who had regular menses, and this may have affected the statistical analyses.

Risk of multiple stress fractures also seems to be increased for athletes who have menstrual disturbance.[42,82] Clark *et al.*[82] found that although groups of amenorrheic and eumenorrheic runners reported a similar prevalence of single stress fractures, 50% of the amenorrheic runners reported multiple stress fractures, compared with only 9% of the runners who were menstruating regularly. For female distance runners, the amenorrheic group was the only group that had a runner who had sustained six stress fractures, whereas for the 120 eumenorrheic runners, no runner had more than three stress fractures.[42]

Grimston and colleagues[89] developed a menstrual index in which previous and current menstrual status was summarized. In the

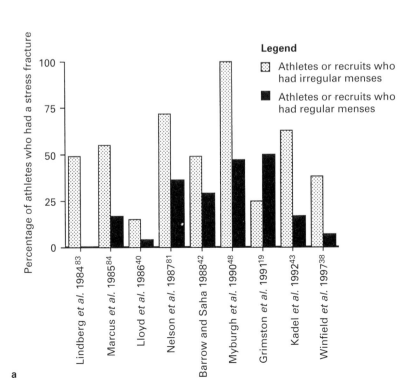

Legend

▨ Athletes or recruits who had irregular menses

■ Athletes or recruits who had regular menses

Percentage of athletes who had a stress fracture (y-axis)

Lindberg *et al.* 1984[83]
Marcus *et al.* 1985[84]
Lloyd *et al.* 1986[40]
Nelson *et al.* 1987[81]
Barrow and Saha 1988[42]
Myburgh *et al.* 1990[48]
Grimston *et al.* 1991[19]
Kadel *et al.* 1992[43]
Winfield *et al.* 1997[38]

a

Fig. 3.5a

The studies in which the percentage of athletes or recruits who had a stress fracture could be compared in groups the members of which had and did not have menstrual irregularity.

Figure 3.5b overleaf.

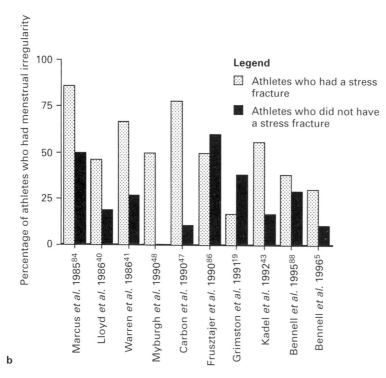

Fig. 3.5b
The studies in which the percentage of athletes or recruits who had menstrual irregularity could be compared in groups the members of which had and did not have a stress fracture.

index, the average number of menses per year since menarche was quantified. Among sixteen female runners, the researchers found no relationship between the menstrual index and stress-fracture incidence. Conversely, track and field athletes who had a lower menstrual index, which indicates fewer menses per year since menarche, were at greater risk of stress fracture compared with athletes who had a higher index.[5] Barrow and Saha[42] also found that lifetime menstrual history affects stress-fracture risk. They revealed that stress-fracture incidence was 29% in the regular-menses group, and 49% in the very-irregular-menses group.

Although it is difficult to make a direct comparison of results because of methodological differences, it would seem that incidence of menstrual disturbances is higher among female athletes who have a stress fracture than in the ones who do not. Some researchers have been led

to assume that these findings are a direct result of a lowered estrogen level and decreased bone-mineral density among athletes who have a menstrual disturbance. However, athletes who have a menstrual disturbance also exhibit other risk factors, such as lower calcium intake,[66] greater training load,[90] and differences in soft-tissue composition.[68] Because these risk factors were not always controlled for in the studies under discussion, it is difficult to ascertain which factors are the contributory ones.

Menstrual disturbances may also predispose female recruits to stress fractures. In a recent prospective cohort study of 101 female Marines, stress-fracture incidence among the women who had fewer than 10 periods per year was 37.5%, compared with 6.7% among the women who had 10 to 13 periods per year.[38] Conversely, in a study of 49 female soldiers who had a stress fracture and 78 soldiers who had no orthopedic injuries, menstrual patterns did not differ between the groups.[45] However, the number of soldiers who had a menstrual disturbance was relatively low.

Given the association between menstrual irregularity and stress-fracture risk, it is important that physically active females be questioned about their current and past menstrual status and that they then seek appropriate medical opinion, if necessary. Because menstrual disturbances are often found together with eating disorders and osteopenia (the three factors are commonly referred to as the 'female-athlete triad'), presence of one of the factors should alert the practitioner to the possibility of presence of the other two.

THE RELATIONSHIP BETWEEN USE OF THE ORAL CONTRACEPTIVE PILL AND STRESS FRACTURES

Some researchers have claimed that use of the oral contraceptive pill (OCP) may protect against stress-fracture development because the OCP provides an exogenous source of estrogen for reducing the remodeling rate and improving bone quality and/or density. No randomized intervention trials have been conducted in order to show that use of the OCP reduces the stress-fracture rate among athletes, particularly among athletes who have or have had a menstrual disturbance.

Two prospective cohort studies – one among athletes,[5] and one among female Marines[38] – failed to support a protective effect of OCP use on stress-fracture development although numbers in the stress-fracture groups were relatively small.

The results of cross-sectional studies are contradictory. Barrow and Saha[42] found that compared with non-users of the OCP (29%), runners who had used the OCP for at least one year had significantly fewer stress fractures (12%). This finding was supported by the findings of Myburgh *et al.*[48] Conversely, no difference in OCP use was reported for ballet dancers some of whom had and some of whom did not have a stress fracture;[43] however, few of the dancers were taking the OCP. Because these studies are retrospective in nature, it is not known whether or not the athletes were taking the OCP before or after the stress fracture occurred. Also, athletes may or may not take the OCP for reasons that in themselves could influence stress-fracture risk. For athletes who have a menstrual disturbance and who subsequently take the OCP, it is not known whether or not stress-fracture risk is decreased.

THE RELATIONSHIP BETWEEN TESTOSTERONE LEVEL AND STRESS FRACTURES IN MALE ATHLETES

The relationship of testosterone levels to bone density and stress-fracture risk in young male athletes has not been well researched. However, in the results of a limited number of studies among male athletes, a relationship between a lowered circulating-testosterone level and osteopenia has failed to be established.[91–93] In a case report, there is a description of the clinical features of a 29-year-old male distance runner who presented with a pelvic stress fracture, markedly decreased bone density, and symptomatic hypogonadotropic hypogonadism.[94] Using this case as an index, the researchers hypothesized that in male athletes, exercise-induced hypogonadotropic hypogonadism can be identified through presence of one or more specific risk factors, which include presence of sexual dysfunction, a history of fracture, and initiation of endurance exercise before eighteen years of age.[95] The researchers compared the levels of free testosterone and luteinizing hormone in fifteen male runners who had one or more of the abovementioned risk factors with the levels of thirteen runners who had none of the risk factors. In the first group, only one of the runners was identified as having primary hypogonadism, and for hormone levels there was no significant difference between the two groups. However, in the runners, bone density was neither measured nor correlated with the testosterone levels.

From a clinical perspective, it is important it be clarified that although some male athletes do present with a reduced testosterone level the concentration usually remains within the normal range for adult men. Therefore, stress-fracture risk may not be increased, and detrimental effects on bone density may not be as dramatic as the effects described for female athletes who have amenorrhea, in which the estradiol level is well below normal.

MENARCHEAL AGE

Menarche is attained later in athletes, especially in sports such as ballet, gymnastics, and running.[96,97] The relationship between menarcheal age and stress-fracture risk is unclear. Some researchers have found that athletes who have a stress fracture have a later menarcheal age,[5,41,47,87] whereas others have found no difference.[43,48,86] In a prospective cohort study, menarcheal age was an independent risk factor for stress fracture among female track and field athletes, and the risk increased by a factor of 4.1 for every additional year of age at menarche[5] (Fig. 3.6).

An association between delayed menarche and stress fractures may be the result of a lower rate of bone-mineral accretion during adolescence, which leads to decreased peak bone mass.[98,99] However, for female athletes the relationship between menarcheal age and bone density is unclear, and although some researchers have found significant but moderate to weak negative correlations at a number of bone sites,[87,100,101] others have not.[70,102,103] Although these results suggest that for female athletes delayed sexual maturation is not strongly associated with lower bone density, many of the samples have been small, and the influence of confounding variables has not been taken into account. In larger cohorts of healthy adolescents and premenopausal and postmenopausal women, the most common finding is that a later menarcheal age is related to lower bone density.[98,104–107] However, this does not imply that a causal relationship exists, because other factors such as genetic background may be a major determinant of both the variables.

A later menarcheal age has also been found in association with menstrual disturbance, lowered energy intake, decreased body fat or weight, and excessive premenarcheal training.[108,109] All these factors could feasibly influence stress-

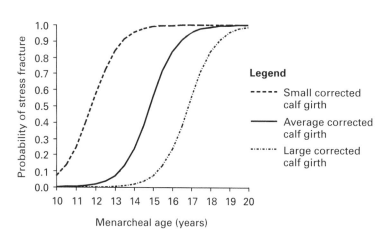

Fig. 3.6

A plot of the probability of stress fracture at various menarcheal ages for various corrected calf girths of female athletes. The plot for small corrected calf girth was calculated by using the minimum value measured in the sample, the average girth was calculated by using the mean value, and the large girth was calculated by using the maximum value. (Source: Adapted and reproduced, with permission, from Bennell *et al.* Risk factors for stress fractures in track and field athletes: a twelve-month prospective study. *American Journal of Sports Medicine* 1996; 24: 810–818.)

fracture risk. Whatever the reason for an association, athletes should be questioned about when their menses commenced. A later menarcheal age could then be used as a marker for identifying a possibly increased risk of fracture.

OTHER HORMONES

Although alterations in calcium metabolism could affect bone remodeling and bone density and therefore predispose a person to stress fracture, no evidence exists that supports this relationship. With reference to military recruits[110] and athletes,[41,47,48] single measurements of serum calcium, parathyroid hormone, 25 OH-vitamin D, and 1,25-dihydroxyvitamin D did not differ between the groups that had and did not have stress fracture. These findings may reflect the sampling procedures, because single measurements were taken at some time point after the stress fracture occurred. Conversely, because many of these biochemical parameters are tightly regulated, alterations in calcium metabolism may not be a factor in stress-fracture development among healthy people. Other endocrine factors that have the potential to influence bone health and therefore stress-fracture risk are glucocorticoids, growth hormone, and thyroxin.

Nutritional factors

Dietary surveys of various sporting groups often reveal inadequate intakes of macronutrients and micronutrients. This is particularly true for females and in sports in which low weight is desirable, such as gymnastics, ballet, and distance running. Presence of abnormal eating behaviors, including disorders such as anorexia nervosa and bulimia nervosa, will also contribute to inadequate dietary intake, and seem to be more common among athletes in specific sports.[67]

Dietary deficiencies, especially dietary-calcium deficiency, may contribute to stress-fracture development by influencing bone density and bone remodeling. In animal studies, a calcium-deficient diet decreases bone's ability to adapt to mechanical strain,[111] whereas high dietary-calcium intake has a favorable effect on bone's biomechanical properties.[112] In some human studies, a positive relationship has been found between dietary-calcium intake and bone mass,[113,114] whereas in others, small bone-mass gains have been noted following calcium supplementation.[115,116]

Because of the following factors, it is difficult to clarify diet's role in bone health and stress-fracture development.

- Accurate assessment of habitual dietary intake is problematic.
- Nutrients may exert their effects on bone over a number of years, so measurement of current intake may not represent lifetime status.
- Calcium balance is negatively influenced by other dietary factors, including high intake of salt, phosphorus, fiber, protein, caffeine, and alcohol.
- Calcium operates as a threshold nutrient, whereby intakes above a certain level produce no additional effects on bone.[117]
- Recommended daily allowances for calcium differ across the lifespan, and the specific needs of physically active people and female athletes who have a menstrual disturbance may not be adequately addressed in them.

The only randomized intervention study in which calcium intake's relationship to stress-fracture development has been assessed was conducted among military recruits. Schwellnus and Jordaan[118] found a similar incidence of stress fractures during a nine-week training program for 247 male recruits who were having a 500 milligram calcium supplement daily, and in 1151 controls who were not taking additional calcium. This result does not seem to support a role for calcium in stress-fracture prevention.

However, nine weeks is probably not long enough for any effects of calcium to become apparent, particularly at cortical lower-limb sites, at which the bone-turnover rate is slower. Furthermore, both groups had a baseline dietary-calcium intake that was greater than 800 milligrams per day, which is the recommended daily allowance for adults. This intake may have been sufficient for protecting against stress fracture, and additional calcium may have provided no added benefit. The effect of calcium supplementation on stress-fracture incidence among people whose usual dietary-calcium intake is below the recommended daily allowance has not been evaluated in any studies.

In a recent cross-sectional study among female military recruits, a difference in dietary-calcium intake was not found between the stress-fracture groups and the non-stress-fracture groups,[45] and this confirms the results of the previously discussed intervention study among male recruits.

For athletes, scant evidence exists that shows that lower calcium intake is associated with increased stress-fracture risk. In a cross-sectional study, Myburgh *et al.*[119] found a significantly lower calcium intake among athletes who had shin soreness, compared with that of a matched control group. However, because exact diagnoses were not made, stress fracture may not have been the only pathology included in the shin-soreness group. A follow-up study among athletes who had a scintigraphically confirmed stress fracture revealed similar results.[48] Current calcium intake was significantly lower in the stress-fracture group: 87% of the recommended daily intake.

In other studies among athletes, a relationship between stress fractures and current dietary-calcium intake has failed to be confirmed.[5,19,43,47,86,87] It was found that ballet dancers consume less than the recommended daily allowance for calcium regardless of their stress-fracture status,[43,86] which implies that for dancers, other factors may be more important as risk factors. For male and female track and field athletes, calcium intake, which was assessed by using four-day food records as well as food-frequency questionnaires, was similar among the athletes who had and did not have a stress fracture.[5] This result does not necessarily exclude calcium deficiency as a risk factor for stress fracture, because most of the athletes in the study were consuming more than the recommended daily allowance of 800 milligrams per day and would therefore not be considered to be calcium deficient.

The relationship of historical calcium intake to stress-fracture occurrence has been evaluated in only one study.[19] A calcium index, based on the variability in calcium intake that occurs between the ages of twelve and twenty-three years, was found to be similar among runners who had and did not have a stress fracture.

Negative influences on calcium balance can include a high intake of salt, protein, phosphorus, fiber, caffeine, and alcohol. At the time of writing, there were no reports of any associations between these nutrients and stress-fracture incidence among athletes.[5,47,48,86,87]

Dietary behaviors and eating patterns may differ among people who have a stress fracture. Ballet dancers who have a stress fracture were more likely to restrict their caloric intake, to avoid high-fat dairy foods, to consume low-calorie products, to have a self-reported history of an eating disorder, and to have a lower percentage of ideal body weight, compared with dancers who did not have a stress fracture.[86]

Similarly, in a cross-sectional study of young-adult, female track and field athletes, the athletes who had a history of stress fracture scored higher on the EAT-40 test (a validated test related to dieting, bulimia and food preoccupation, and oral control), and compared with the athletes who did not have a stress fracture were more likely to engage in restrictive eating patterns and dieting.[88] For the same group when it was followed prospectively, four-day food records revealed a lower-fat diet among the females who went on to develop a stress fracture during the year of the study.[5] More recently, a large multicenter survey of 2298 United States collegiate athletes revealed that the White females who had a history of pathogenic weight-control behaviors had a 1.96 relative-odds ratio for having a stress fracture, compared with the athletes who did not have this history.[67] These studies suggest that disordered eating patterns are associated with higher risk for stress fracture. It is not clear whether this association is causal or the result of some other factor.

In summary, at present, not much evidence exists that supports dietary deficiencies, especially low calcium intake, as being a risk factor in otherwise healthy recreational and elite athletes and military recruits. Conversely, abnormal and restrictive eating behaviors do seem to be related to greater likelihood of fracture. Healthy eating habits should be promoted for all people. If the practitioner is concerned about dietary intake among athletes, food records as well as biochemical and anthropometric indices can be used for assessing dietary adequacy and nutritional status.

Physical training

Repetitive mechanical loading that arises from athletics training contributes to stress-fracture development. However, the contribution of each training component (type, volume, intensity, frequency, and rate of change) to stress-fracture risk has not been elucidated. Training may also influence bone indirectly, through changes in levels of circulating hormones, through effects on soft-tissue composition, and through associations with menstrual disturbances.

PHYSICAL FITNESS

It is unclear whether or not lack of prior physical activity and poor physical conditioning predispose a person to stress fracture, because many groups of researchers have relied on self-reporting rather than standardized fitness tests before the exercise program was commenced. In most of the literature, the focus is on military recruits who are subjected to a short burst of intensive, unaccustomed activity, and who are often unfit.

In some military studies, a correlation between self-reported previous physical-activity levels and stress-fracture rate during basic training has been reported, whereas in others a relationship has failed to be corroborated. Montgomery *et al.*[29] found that male trainees who had a running history and who averaged at least 25 miles per week in the previous year had a lower incidence of stress fracture (3%), compared with trainees who averaged fewer than four miles per week (11.5%). Similarly, Gardner *et al.*[120] found the stress-fracture rate to be twenty-four times greater in the previously inactive group than in the very active group. In a prospective cohort study among female United States Marines, the women who reported running less than 2.8 miles per session had a 16.3% stress-fracture incidence during basic training, compared with 3.8% of the women who ran more than 2.8 miles per session.[38] However, no relationship was found between stress fractures and frequency of running sessions or between stress fractures and a battery of fitness tests, including running, sit-ups, and push-ups. In a study of female United States military recruits, the researchers reported that higher leisure-activity energy expenditure tended to be associated with lower stress-fracture risk ($P = 0.06$).[45]

Conversely, in the largest study, neither aerobic fitness, measured by calculating the predicted VO_2max, nor self-reported pretraining participation in sport activities was related to stress-fracture incidence among 295 male recruits between 18 and 20 years of age.[121] This lack of association was confirmed in another large study of 270 male recruits by using predicted VO_2max.[15]

Although the data are conflicting, the larger prospective studies tend to suggest that physical fitness is not a predictor of stress-fracture risk for people who are undergoing basic military training. Poor physical conditioning does not seem to apply to athletes, because stress fractures often occur in well-conditioned people who have been training for years.

TRAINING REGIMEN

Aspects of the training regimen can influence stress-fracture development. Military studies have shown that various training modifications can decrease stress-fracture incidence among recruits. These interventions include rest periods,[122,123] elimination of running and marching on concrete,[124,125] use of running shoes instead of combat boots,[125,126] and reduction of high-impact activity.[44,123,127] These interventions may reduce stress-fracture risk by providing time for bone microdamage to be repaired and by decreasing the load applied to bone.

By contrast, there is not much controlled research among athletes. Most of the research comprises either anecdotal observations or case-series in which training parameters are examined only for the athletes who have a stress fracture. For example, in surveys in which it is reported that up to 86% of athletes can identify some change in their training before the onset of the stress fracture,[31,128] a similar comparison for uninjured athletes is not provided. Other researchers have blamed training 'errors' in a varying proportion of cases, but they do not adequately define the 'errors'.[30,129–131] Brunet *et al.*[37] surveyed 1505 runners, and found that increasing mileage correlated with increase in stress fractures among women but not among men. It is unclear how the apparent gender difference can be explained. In a study of ballet dancers, a dancer who trained for more than five hours per day had an estimated stress-fracture risk that was sixteen times greater than that of a dancer who trained for less than five

hours per day.[43] These studies support a role for training volume as being a risk factor for stress fracture.

It is evident that bone remodeling is able to repair microdamage if given adequate time, but that a stress fracture results if a load is repeatedly applied. It would therefore be surmised that cyclic training is preferable to progressive training in order to enable both bone and soft tissue to rest from repetitive loading. Athletes and military personnel should undertake alternative aerobic exercise that includes low-impact loading for a week after two to three weeks of training. Furthermore, exercise such as cycling or swimming should be added to the weekly training regimen in place of running.

In the clinical setting, it is imperative that a detailed training history be obtained in order to try and identify any training parameters that may have contributed to the person's stress fracture. Questions should especially be directed at establishing volume, intensity, extent of rest periods, type of training, and any recent changes in these parameters. Furthermore, athletes should be encouraged to keep an accurate log book for their training. This will enable them to monitor their training and to gauge the appropriateness of any training changes. They should be counseled about the nature of overuse injuries, and should be advised to seek medical assistance at the first onset of any pain. If overuse is identified early in the continuum, a period of reduced activity may break the cycle and enable a stress reaction to heal rather than develop into an actual stress fracture.

Extrinsic mechanical factors

SURFACE

Training surface has long been considered to be a contributor to stress-fracture development.[132] Anatomic and biomechanical problems can be accentuated through use of cambered or uneven surfaces, and ground-reaction forces are increased through use of less compliant surfaces.[133,134] Alternatively, running on softer surfaces may hasten muscle fatigue. In large epidemiological studies of overall running injuries an association between injury and training surface or terrain has failed to be shown after controlling for the effects of weekly running distance.[135,136] However, this may be related to the difficulty involved in accurately quantifying running-surface parameters, and to the difficulty involved in sampling bias. Although no data exist whereby the relationship of training surface and stress fractures is specifically assessed, it may be prudent to advise athletes to minimize the time they spend training on hard, uneven surfaces.

FOOTWEAR, INSOLES AND ORTHOTICS

For athletic footwear, insoles and orthotics, the aim is to attenuate shock when ground contact is made and to control the motion of the foot and ankle. The material characteristics and construction of a shoe's midsole mainly determine the shoe's shock-absorbing and attenuating properties.[137] By using price as a surrogate measure of the quality of running shoes, the research group in a large prospective study failed to find a significant difference in stress-fracture rates among recruits who were wearing high-quality runners, compared with recruits who were wearing low-quality runners.[120] However, the assumption that price equates with quality is not necessarily valid. A shoe's age is believed to provide an indication of the midsole's condition. In the same study, a significantly higher stress-fracture rate was found among recruits who were wearing older or worn running shoes.[120] Although for older shoes this finding could be the result of decreased shock absorption, age also has a detrimental effect on the mechanical support that the shoe provides.[138] Similar results were reported in a study of twenty-five patients who had shin

soreness and twenty-five matched controls, whereby 80% of the injured subjects were wearing worn shoes, compared with 44% of the controls.[119]

Changing from military boots to athletic shoes may reduce incidence of stress fractures in the foot.[125,139] An experimental study was conducted among 390 infantry recruits in order to evaluate whether or not incidence of overuse injuries was affected by footwear type.[139] Basketball shoes were provided to 187 randomly selected recruits, and the rest of the recruits wore standard military boots. After fourteen weeks of basic training, no significant difference was found between overall stress-fracture rates among the two footwear groups. However, the recruits who trained in basketball shoes had a significantly lower incidence of overuse injuries of the foot, which suggests that the effect may be limited to injuries that result from vertical-impact loads. Injuries such as tibial stress fractures, which are secondary to bending forces, were not affected by use of a more cushioned shoe.[137] However, the results of a pilot study in which rosette strain gauges were mounted on to a human subject's tibial mid shaft revealed that shoe type can influence tibial strains during walking and running.[140] Surprisingly, in this study a new form of infantry boot produced the lowest compressive strains, compared with various sport shoes, despite the boot's relatively high weight and sole durometry.

Shock-absorbing insoles are often used in an attempt to reduce incidence of overuse injuries. Many types of insole are on the market, and they vary in their ability to both absorb shock and change foot biomechanics. For example, Cinats et al.[141] found that use of Sorbothane inserts reduced the final transmitted stress over the duration of heel strike by less than 10%, and Voloshin and Wosk[142] found that viscoelastic inserts reduced shock-wave amplitudes during gait by an average of forty-two. Reports are conflicting about whether or not insoles can prevent stress fracture.

An animal model was used to assess the effect of viscoelastic orthotics on incidence of tibial stress fracture.[143] The hindlimbs of skeletally mature rabbits were passively loaded for five days per week over a six- or nine-week period. Tibial stress fractures were sustained by 90% of the rabbits that trained using orthotics and by 92% of the rabbits that trained using orthotics.

In a randomized experimental study among Israeli Army recruits, although use of a semirigid orthotic device made no significant difference to overall incidence of stress fractures during basic training, it did reduce incidence of femoral stress fractures.[144] It is unclear why an insole effect was limited to only femoral stress fractures. When the data were analyzed in more detail, an interaction seemed to occur between foot type, the orthotic, and the stress-fracture site.[27] For recruits who wore the orthotic, incidence of femoral stress fractures was reduced for the people who had high-arched feet, and incidence of metatarsal fractures was reduced for the people who had low-arched feet. Incidence of tibial stress fractures was not affected by use of this orthotic device. Because the device had a hindfoot post at 3° varus that altered the foot's biomechanics, it is difficult to know whether the study's results can be attributed to this feature or to the shock-absorption capability.

In another large intervention study of 3025 United States Marines, no difference was found between the stress-fracture rate among the experimental-group members who wore the viscoelastic polymer insole, and the control group.[120] This contrasts with the results of a similar study among South African recruits, in which 250 recruits wore neoprene insoles in their shoes during nine weeks of basic training, and 1151 recruits acted as controls.[145] Compliance was good: 85% of the recruits reported that they wore the insoles daily. The results showed that the insoles significantly reduced overall incidence of overuse injuries and that there was a noticeable trend for stress fractures (0% in the experimental group, and 1.4% in the control

group). The difference in results may be because of differences in the insoles. It has been shown that viscoelastic insoles do not significantly reduce vertical-impact forces when compared with conventional running-shoe insoles.[146] Furthermore, it has been found that neoprene insoles are less rigid, are more resistant to shear-compression forces, and are better able to reduce transmitted force, compared with viscoelastic insoles.[147]

For track and field athletes, clinical observation suggests that use of running spikes may influence likelihood of stress fracture. At the time of writing, there was insufficient research into the relationship of this form of footwear and risk of stress-fracture development.

From a practical point of view, it is important that individuals train in shoes that are appropriate for their foot type. When an athlete is selecting a shoe, the important features he or she should consider are midsole hardness, midsole width, heel flare, heel height, stability devices, and torsional flexibility (Fig. 3.7). Athletes who have high arches should consider shock-absorbing features to be a priority, whereas athletes who have low arches require support for excessive motion.

EXTERNAL LOADING

In humans, direct measurement of bone strain by way of surgical attachment of a bone-strain gauge has both ethical and methodological constraints. Ground-reaction force (GRF), which is measured by way of a force platform set into the floor, can provide an indirect measure of both the magnitude and the rate of external load on the lower extremity during physical activity.[148]

For predicting stress-fracture risk, evidence is conflicting about the role of external loading as measured by way of GRF. In two cross-sectional studies, Grimston and colleagues[19,64] found significant differences in GRF, during running, between the stress-fracture and non-stress-fracture groups. However, in their initial study,

Upper: This is the shoe part that covers the foot. The toe box, which is usually covered by the wing tip – a leather overlay – is located at the front of the upper, and must provide adequate room for the toes' dorsiflexion and plantarflexion. Some shoes have reinforcement of the medial arch by way of a saddle (outside) or an arch bandage (inside). The tongue provides protection from the laces by covering the foot's dorsum. The heel counter is designed to cradle the heel in order to stabilize the subtalar joint and to help control excessive pronation. It must be rigid yet comfortable around the Achilles-tendon region.

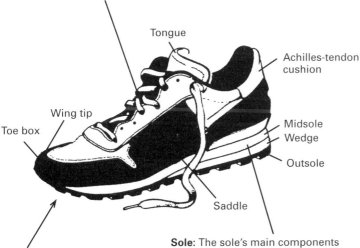

Tongue

Achilles-tendon cushion

Wing tip

Midsole
Wedge

Toe box

Outsole

Saddle

Foot shape: This is either straight lasted or curve lasted, and the straight last provides greater medial support. Board lasting or slip lasting is the way in which the shoe's upper part is attached to the sole. In board lasting, the upper is attached to a hard, fibrous inner-sole board. The shoe is often heavier but provides more stability and is therefore suited to heavier runners or people who overpronate. In slip lasting, the upper is stitched into a one-piece moccasin that is then glued into a pre-cut sole. The shoe is often lighter, roomier in the toe box and more flexible and is therefore suited to people who have cavus feet.

Sole: The sole's main components are the outsole, midsole, and wedge. The outsole is designed for traction and shock absorption and should be durable. The midsole is the main shock absorber. It comes in varying densities that are used in combination to dissipate shock and to control pronation. It runs the length of the shoe, and should be flexible. The wedge acts as a heel lift, and also provides shock absorption. Although heel flare's angle has been varied, a wide flare is not recommended, because in some runners it has been implicated in pain development. The heel's height varies. The heel of training shoes is higher than that of racing flats, because the extra height increases the shoe's ability to absorb shock, and reduces strain on the Achilles tendon.

Fig. 3.7

Important features to consider when a training shoe is being selected. (Source: Adapted from McKenzie DC, Clement DB, Taunton JE. Running shoes, orthotics, and injuries. *Sports Medicine* 1985; 2: 334–347.)

the forces were higher in the stress-fracture group, whereas in the subsequent study they were lower. Sample characteristics and testing procedures differed between their two studies, and in some aspects were not well controlled, which may have contributed to the inconsistent findings. In particular, the samples were small and heterogeneous, there was an insufficient number of running trials, and the running speed was not standardized. In a more recent and larger cross-sectional study among forty-six male runners, a role for external-loading kinetics in stress-fracture development was failed to be supported.[16]

Other factors

GENETIC PREDISPOSITION

Twin studies have indicated that between 40% and 90% of the variation in bone mass can be attributed to genetic factors.[149] Not surprisingly, therefore, a family history of osteoporosis is considered to be a risk factor for low bone density and osteoporosis in both men and women.[150,151] The exact mechanism for this strong genetic influence on bone density is unknown, and controversy currently exists about the role of Vitamin D receptor-gene alleles.[152]

It is feasible that some people may be genetically predisposed to stress fractures when exposed to suitable environmental conditions, such as vigorous exercise, although few data exist for evaluating the role of genetic factors in predisposing an athlete to stress fracture. Existence of a case report in which identical multiple stress fractures were sustained in femoral and tarsal bones by a pair of eighteen-year-old monozygotic twins who were undergoing basic military training does imply a possible genetic predisposition.[153] Myburgh *et al.*[48] failed to find a difference in incidence of a family history of osteoporosis among athletes who had and did not have stress fracture.

PSYCHOLOGICAL TRAITS

Not much information exists about psychological traits and stress fractures, particularly with reference to athletes. Of the three prospective studies conducted in the military, two research groups failed to find an association between psychological factors and stress-fracture incidence. Pretraining motivation, assessed by way of the Quality Index, was not related to the 31% stress-fracture incidence among male Israeli military recruits.[15] Similarly, Taimela *et al.*[44] found that in multivariate analysis, stress fractures could not be predicted by way of psychomotor reaction-time parameters, mental-ability parameters, and specific personality traits. Conversely, low-achievement and high-obedience personality traits were related to increased incidence of stress fractures among 108 army conscripts.[154] However, these results may not be extrapolated directly to athletes who are involved in voluntary exercise. It could be speculated that instead, high achievement and motivation may be related to greater training volume and intensity, and perhaps to disordered eating patterns, all of which could contribute to stress-fracture development.

SUMMARY

- Although most studies in which the risk factors associated with stress-fracture development have been evaluated do not enable causality to be assigned, several important insights can be gleaned from the existing literature.
- Although it falls short of proving that menstrual disturbances, caloric restriction, low bone density, muscle weakness, and leg-length differences are contributory factors, the literature indicates that it is wise to pursue evidence of these factors clinically, and to adjust treatment accordingly.
- Likewise, although time-honored risk factors such as lower-extremity alignment and training factors (volume, intensity, and surface) have not yet been shown to be causative, anecdotal evidence indicates that they are likely to have an important role in stress-fracture pathogenesis.

References

1 Lysens RJ, de Weerdt W, Nieuwboer A. Factors associated with injury proneness. *Sports Medicine* 1991; 12: 281–289.

2 Meeuwisse WH. Athletic injury etiology: distinguishing between interaction and confounding. *Clinical Journal of Sport Medicine* 1994; 4: 171–175.

3 Schootman M, Powell JW, Torner JC. Study designs and potential biases in sports injury research: the case-control study. *Sports Medicine* 1994; 18: 22–37.

4 Walter SD, Sutton JR, McIntosh JM, Connolly C. The aetiology of sports injuries: a review of methodologies. *Sports Medicine* 1985; 2: 47–58.

5 Bennell KL, Malcolm SA, Thomas SA *et al.* Risk factors for stress fractures in track and field athletes: a 12 month prospective study. *American Journal of Sports Medicine* 1996; 24: 810–818.

6 van Mechelen W, Hlobil H, Kemper HCG. Incidence, severity, aetiology and prevention of sports injuries: a review of concepts. *Sports Medicine* 1992; 14: 82–99.

7 Meeuwisse WH. Assessing causation in sport injury: a multifactorial model. *Clinical Journal of Sport Medicine* 1994; 4: 166–170.

8 Carter DR, Caler WE, Spengler DM, Frankel VH. Uniaxial fatigue of human cortical bone: the influence of tissue physical characteristics. *Journal of Biomechanics* 1981; 14: 461–470.

9 Cummings SR, Black DM, Nevitt MC *et al.* Bone density at various sites for prediction of hip fractures. *Lancet* 1993; 341: 72–75.

10 Melton LJ, Atkinson EJ, O'Fallon WM, Wahner HW, Riggs BL. Long-term fracture prediction by bone mineral assessed at different skeletal sites. *Journal of Bone and Mineral Research* 1993; 8: 1227–1233.

11 Wark JD. Bone density measurement. *Australian Prescriber* 1992; 15: 62–65.

12 Mazess RB, Barden HS, Bisek JP, Hanson J. Dual-energy x-ray absorptiometry for total-body and regional bone-mineral and soft-tissue composition. *American Journal of Clinical Nutrition* 1990; 51: 1106–1112.

13 Johnson J, Dawson-Hughes B. Precision and stability of dual-energy x-ray absorptiometry measurements. *Calcified Tissue International* 1991; 49: 174–178.

14 Russell-Aulet M, Wang J, Thornton J, Pierson RN. Comparison of dual-photon absorptiometry system for total-body bone and soft tissue measurements: dual-energy x-rays versus gadolinium-153. *Journal of Bone and Mineral Research* 1991; 6: 411–415.

15 Giladi M, Milgrom C, Simkin A, Danon Y. Stress fractures: identifiable risk factors. *American Journal of Sports Medicine* 1991; 19: 647–652.

16 Crossley K, Bennell KL, Wrigley T, Oakes BW. Ground reaction forces, bone characteristics and tibial stress fracture in male runners. *Medicine and Science in Sports and Exercise* 1999. (In press.)

17 Beck TJ, Ruff CB, Mourtada FA *et al.* Dual-energy x-ray absorptiometry derived structural geometry for stress fracture prediction in male U.S. Marine Corps recruits. *Journal of Bone and Mineral Research* 1996; 11: 645–653.

18 Pouilles JM, Bernard J, Tremollieres F, Louvet JP, Ribot C. Femoral bone density in young male adults with stress fractures. *Bone* 1989; 10: 105–108.

19 Grimston SK, Engsberg JR, Kloiber R, Hanley DA. Bone mass, external loads, and stress fractures in female runners. *International Journal of Sport Biomechanics* 1991; 7: 293–302.

20 Nordin M, Frankel VH. *Basic Biomechanics of the Musculoskeletal System*, 5th edn. Philadelphia: Lea and Febiger, 1989.

21 Miller GJ, Purkey WW. The geometric properties of paired human tibiae. *Journal of Biomechanics* 1980; 13: 1–8.

22 Martens M, Van Auderkerke R, de Meester P, Mulier JC. The geometrical properties of human femur and tibia and their importance for the mechanical behaviour of these bone structures. *Acta Orthopaedica Traumatica Surgery* 1981; 98: 113–120.

23 Giladi M, Milgrom C, Simkin A *et al.* Stress fractures and tibial bone width: a risk factor. *Journal of Bone and Joint Surgery* 1987; 69-B: 326–329.

24 Milgrom C, Giladi M, Simkin A *et al.* An analysis of the biomechanical mechanism of tibial stress fractures among Israeli infantry recruits. *Clinical Orthopaedics and Related Research* 1988; 231: 216–221.

25 Milgrom C, Giladi M, Simkin A *et al.* The area moment of inertia of the tibia: a risk factor for stress fractures. *Journal of Biomechanics* 1989; 22: 1243–1248.

26 Giladi M, Milgrom C, Stein M *et al.* The low arch, a protective factor in stress fractures: a prospective study of 295 military recruits. *Orthopaedic Review* 1985; 14: 709–712.

27 Simkin A, Leichter I, Giladi M, Stein M, Milgrom C. Combined effect of foot arch structure and an orthotic device on stress fractures. *Foot and Ankle* 1989; 10: 25–29.

28 Brosh T, Arcan M. Toward early detection of the tendency to stress fractures. *Clinical Biomechanics* 1994; 9: 111–116.

29 Montgomery LC, Nelson FRT, Norton JP, Deuster FA. Orthopedic history and examination in the etiology of overuse injuries. *Medicine and Science in Sports and Exercise* 1989; 21: 237–243.

30 Taunton JE, Clement DB, Webber D. Lower extremity stress fractures in athletes. *Physician and Sportsmedicine* 1981; 9: 77–86.

31 Sullivan D, Warren RF, Pavlov H, Kelman G. Stress fractures in 51 runners. *Clinical Orthopaedics and Related Research* 1984; 187: 188–192.

32 Matheson GO, Clement DB, McKenzie DC *et al*. Stress fractures in athletes: a study of 320 cases. *American Journal of Sports Medicine* 1987; 15: 46–58.

33 Ekenman I, Tsai-Fellander L, Westblad P, Turan I, Rolf C. A study of intrinsic factors in patients with stress fractures of the tibia. *Foot and Ankle International* 1996; 17: 477–482.

34 D'Amico JC, Dinowitz HD, Polchaninoff M. Limb length discrepancy: an electrodynographic analysis. *Journal of the American Podiatry Medical Association* 1985; 75: 639–643.

35 Cowan DN, Jones BH, Frykman PN *et al*. Lower limb morphology and risk of overuse injury among male infantry trainees. *Medicine and Science in Sports and Exercise* 1996; 28: 945–952.

36 Friberg O. Leg length asymmetry in stress fractures: a clinical and radiological study. *Journal of Sports Medicine* 1982; 22: 485–488.

37 Brunet ME, Cook SD, Brinker MR, Dickinson JA. A survey of running injuries in 1505 competitive and recreational runners. *Journal of Sports Medicine and Physical Fitness* 1990; 30: 307–315.

38 Winfield AC, Bracker M, Moore J, Johnson CW. Risk factors associated with stress reactions in female marines. *Military Medicine* 1997; 162: 698–702.

39 Frederick EC, Hagy JL. Factors affecting peak vertical ground reaction forces in running. *International Journal of Sport Biomechanics* 1986; 2: 41–49.

40 Lloyd T, Triantafyllou SJ, Baker ER *et al*. Women athletes with menstrual irregularity have increased musculoskeletal injuries. *Medicine and Science in Sports and Exercise* 1986; 18: 374–379.

41 Warren MP, Brooks-Gunn J, Hamilton LH, Warren LF, Hamilton WG. Scoliosis and fractures in young ballet dancers. *New England Journal of Medicine* 1986; 314: 1348–1353.

42 Barrow GW, Saha S. Menstrual irregularity and stress fractures in collegiate female distance runners. *American Journal of Sports Medicine* 1988; 16: 209–216.

43 Kadel NJ, Teitz CC, Kronmal RA. Stress fractures in ballet dancers. *American Journal of Sports Medicine* 1992; 20: 445–449.

44 Taimela S, Kujala UM, Dahlstrom S, Koskinen S. Risk factors for stress fractures during physical training programs. *Clinical Journal of Sport Medicine* 1992; 2: 105–108.

45 Cline AD, Jansen GR, Melby CL. Stress fractures in female army recruits – implications of bone density, calcium

intake, and exercise. *Journal of the American College of Nutrition* 1998; 17: 128–135.

46 Murguia MJ, Vailas A, Mandelbaum B *et al*. Elevated plasma hydroxyproline: a possible risk factor associated with connective tissue injuries during overuse. *American Journal of Sports Medicine* 1988; 16: 660–664.

47 Carbon R, Sambrook PN, Deakin V *et al*. Bone density of elite female athletes with stress fractures. *Medical Journal of Australia* 1990; 153: 373–376.

48 Myburgh KH, Hutchins J, Fataar AB, Hough SF, Noakes TD. Low bone density is an etiologic factor for stress fractures in athletes. *Annals of Internal Medicine* 1990; 113: 754–759.

49 Bennell KL, Malcolm SA, Brukner PD *et al*. A 12-month prospective study of the relationship between stress fractures and bone turnover in athletes. *Calcified Tissue International* 1998; 63: 80–85.

50 Giladi M, Milgrom C, Stein M *et al*. External rotation of the hip: a predictor of risk for stress fractures. *Clinical Orthopaedics and Related Research* 1987; 216: 131–134.

51 Milgrom C, Finestone A, Shlamkovitch N *et al*. Youth is a risk factor for stress fracture: a study of 783 infantry recruits. *Journal of Bone and Joint Surgery* 1994; 76-B: 20–22.

52 Hughes LY. Biomechanical analysis of the foot and ankle for predisposition to developing stress fractures. *Journal of Orthopaedic and Sports Physical Therapy* 1985; 7: 96–101.

53 Stanitski CL, McMaster JH, Scranton PE. On the nature of stress fractures. *American Journal of Sports Medicine* 1978; 6: 391–396.

54 Meyer SA, Saltzman CL, Albright JP. Stress fractures of the foot and leg. *Clinics in Sports Medicine* 1993; 12: 395–413.

55 Voloshin A, Wosk J. An *in vivo* study of low back pain and shock absorption in the human locomotor system. *Journal of Biomechanics* 1982; 15: 21–27.

56 Cavanagh PR, LaFortune MA. Ground reaction forces in distance running. *Journal of Biomechanics* 1980; 13: 397–406.

57 Bates BT, Osternig LR, Sawhill JA. An assessment of subject variability, subject-shoe interaction, and the evaluation of running shoes using ground reaction force data. *Journal of Biomechanics* 1983; 16: 181–191.

58 McNitt-Gray J. Kinematics and impulse characteristics of drop landings from three heights. *International Journal of Sports Biomechanics* 1991; 7: 201–223.

59 Paul IL, Munro MB, Abernethy PJ *et al*. Musculo-skeletal shock absorption: relative contribution of bone and soft tissues at various frequencies. *Journal of Biomechanics* 1978; 11: 237–239.

60 Clement DB. Tibial stress syndrome in athletes. *Journal of Sports Medicine* 1974; 2: 81–85.

61 Benazzo F, Barnabei G, Ferrario A, Castelli C, Fischetto G. Stress fractures in track and field athletes. *Journal of Sports Traumatology and Related Research* 1992; 14: 51–65.

62 Milgrom C. The Israeli elite infantry recruit: a model for understanding the biomechanics of stress fractures. *Journal of the Royal College of Surgeons Edinburgh* 1989; 34: S18–S22.

63 Scott SH, Winter DA. Internal forces at chronic running injury sites. *Medicine and Science in Sports and Exercise* 1990; 22: 357–369.

64 Grimston SK, Nigg BM, Fisher V, Ajemian SV. External loads throughout a 45 minute run in stress fracture and non-stress fracture runners. *Journal of Biomechanics* 1994; 27: 668.

65 Malina RM, Spriduso WW, Tate C, Baylor AM. Age at menarche and selected menstrual characteristics in athletes at different competitive levels and in different sports. *Medicine and Science in Sports and Exercise* 1978; 10: 218–222.

66 Kaiserauer S, Snyder AC, Sleeper M, Zierath J. Nutritional, physiological, and menstrual status of distance runners. *Medicine and Science in Sports and Exercise* 1989; 21: 120–125.

67 Nattiv A, Puffer JC, Green GA. Lifestyles and health risks of collegiate athletes – a multi-center study. *Clinical Journal of Sport Medicine* 1997; 7: 262–272.

68 Wolman RL, Harries MG. Menstrual abnormalities in elite athletes. *Clinical Sports Medicine* 1989; 1: 95–100.

69 Drinkwater BL, Nilson K, Chesnut III CH *et al.* Bone mineral content of amenorrheic and eumenorrheic athletes. *New England Journal of Medicine* 1984; 5: 277–281.

70 Rutherford OM. Spine and total body bone mineral density in amenorrheic endurance athletes. *Journal of Applied Physiology* 1993; 74: 2904–2908.

71 Micklesfield LK, Lambert EV, Fataar AB, Noakes TD, Myburgh KH. Bone mineral density in mature, premenopausal ultramarathon runners. *Medicine and Science in Sports and Exercise* 1995; 27: 688–696.

72 Tomten SE, Falch JA, Birkeland KI, Hemmersbach P, Hostmark AT. Bone mineral density and menstrual irregularities – a comparative study on cortical and trabecular bone structures in runners with alleged normal eating behaviour. *International Journal of Sports Medicine* 1998; 19: 92–97.

73 Beitins IZ, McArthur JW, Turnbull BA, Skrinar GS, Bullen BA. Exercise induces two types of human luteal dysfunction: confirmation by urinary free progesterone. *Journal of Clinical Endocrinology and Metabolism* 1991; 72: 1350–1358.

74 Prior JC, Vigna YM. Ovulation disturbances and exercise training. *Clinical Obstetrics and Gynecology* 1991; 34: 180–190.

75 Snow GR, Anderson C. The effects of continuous progestogen treatment on cortical bone remodeling activity in beagles. *Calcified Tissue International* 1985; 37: 282–286.

76 Karambolova KK, Snow GR, Anderson C. Surface activity on the periosteal and corticoendosteal envelopes following continuous progestogen supplementation in spayed beagles. *Calcified Tissue International* 1986; 38: 239–243.

77 Snow GR, Anderson C. The effects of 17β-estradiol and progestagen on trabecular bone remodeling in oophorectomized dogs. *Calcified Tissue International* 1986; 39: 198–205.

78 Prior JC, Vigna YM, Schechter MT, Burgess AE. Spinal bone loss and ovulatory disturbances. *New England Journal of Medicine* 1990; 323: 1221–1227.

79 Snead DB, Weltman A, Weltman JY *et al.* Reproductive hormones and bone mineral density in women runners. *Journal of Applied Physiology* 1992; 72: 2149–2156.

80 Barr SI, Prior JC, Vigna YM. Restrained eating and ovulatory disturbances: possible implications for bone health. *American Journal of Clinical Nutrition* 1994; 59: 92–97.

81 Nelson ME, Clark N, Otradovec C, Evans WJ. Elite women runners: association between menstrual status, weight history and stress fractures. *Medicine and Science in Sports and Exercise* 1987; 19: S13.

82 Clark N, Nelson M, Evans W. Nutrition education for elite female runners. *Physician and Sportsmedicine* 1988; 16: 124–136.

83 Lindberg JS, Fears WB, Hunt MM *et al.* Exercise-induced amenorrhea and bone density. *Annals of Internal Medicine* 1984; 101: 647–648.

84 Marcus R, Cann C, Madvig P *et al.* Menstrual function and bone mass in elite women distance runners. *Annals of Internal Medicine* 1985; 102: 158–163.

85 Cook SD, Harding AF, Thomas KA *et al.* Trabecular bone density and menstrual function in women runners. *American Journal of Sports Medicine* 1987; 15: 503–507.

86 Frusztajer NT, Dhuper S, Warren MP, Brooks-Gunn J, Fox RP. Nutrition and the incidence of stress fractures in ballet dancers. *American Journal of Clinical Nutrition* 1990; 51: 779–783.

87 Warren MP, Brooks-Gunn J, Fox RP *et al.* Lack of bone accretion and amenorrhea: evidence for a relative osteopenia in weight bearing bones. *Journal of Clinical Endocrinology and Metabolism* 1991; 72: 847–853.

88 Bennell KL, Malcolm SA, Thomas SA *et al.* Risk factors for stress fractures in female track-and-field athletes: a

retrospective analysis. *Clinical Journal of Sport Medicine* 1995; 5: 229–235.

89 Grimston SK, Engsberg JR, Kloiber R, Hanley DA. Menstrual, calcium, and training history: relationship to bone health in female runners. *Clinical Sports Medicine* 1990; 2: 119–128.

90 Guler F, Hascelik Z. Menstrual dysfunction rate and delayed menarche in top athletes of team games. *Sports Medicine, Training and Rehabilitation* 1993; 4: 99–106.

91 MacDougall JD, Webber CE, Martin J *et al.* Relationship among running mileage, bone density, and serum testosterone in male runners. *Journal of Applied Physiology* 1992; 73: 1165–1170.

92 Hetland ML, Haarbo J, Christiansen C. Low bone mass and high bone turnover in male long distance runners. *Journal of Clinical Endocrinology and Metabolism* 1993; 77: 770–775.

93 Smith R, Rutherford OM. Spine and total body bone mineral density and serum testosterone levels in male athletes. *European Journal of Applied Physiology* 1993; 67: 330–334.

94 Burge MR, Lanzi RA, Skarda ST, Eaton RP. Idiopathic hypogonadotropic hypogonadism in a male runner is reversed by clomiphene citrate. *Fertility and Sterility* 1997; 67: 783–785.

95 Skarda ST, Burge MR. Prospective evaluation of risk factors for exercise-induced hypogonadism in male runners. *Western Journal of Medicine* 1998; 169: 9–12.

96 Malina RM. Menarche in athletes: a synthesis and hypothesis. *Annals of Human Biology* 1983; 10: 1–24.

97 Stager JM, Hatler LK. Menarche in athletes: the influence of genetics and prepubertal training. *Medicine and Science in Sports and Exercise* 1988; 20: 369–373.

98 Lu PW, Briody JN, Ogle GD *et al.* Bone mineral density of total body, spine, and femoral neck in children and young adults: a cross-sectional and longitudinal study. *Journal of Bone and Mineral Research* 1994; 9: 1451–1458.

99 Young D, Hopper JL, Nowson CA *et al.* Determinants of bone mass in 10- to 26-year-old females: a twin study. *Journal of Bone and Mineral Research* 1995; 10: 558–567.

100 Dhuper S, Warren MP, Brooks-Gunn J, Fox R. Effects of hormonal status on bone density in adolescent girls. *Journal of Clinical Endocrinology and Metabolism* 1990; 71: 1083–1088.

101 Robinson TL, Snow-Harter C, Taaffe DR *et al.* Gymnasts exhibit higher bone mass than runners despite similar prevalence of amenorrhea and oligomenorrhea. *Journal of Bone and Mineral Research* 1995; 10: 26–35.

102 Fehily AM, Coles RJ, Evans WD, Elwood PC. Factors affecting bone density in young adults. *American Journal of Clinical Nutrition* 1992; 56: 579–586.

103 Myburgh KH, Bachrach LK, Lewis B, Kent K, Marcus R. Low bone mineral density at axial and appendicular sites in amenorrheic athletes. *Medicine and Science in Sports and Exercise* 1993; 25: 1197–1202.

104 Katzman DK, Bachrach LK, Carter DR, Marcus R. Clinical and anthropometric correlates of bone mineral acquisition in healthy adolescent girls. *Journal of Clinical Endocrinology and Metabolism* 1991; 73: 1332–1339.

105 Armamento-Villareal R, Villareal DT, Avioli LV, Civtelli R. Estrogen status and heredity are major determinants of premenopausal bone loss. *Journal of Clinical Investigations* 1992; 90: 2464–2471.

106 Elliot JR, Gilchrist NL, Wells JE *et al.* Historical assessment of risk factors in screening for osteopenia in a normal Caucasian population. *Australian and New Zealand Journal of Medicine* 1993; 23: 458–462.

107 Fox KM, Magaziner J, Sherwin R *et al.* Reproductive correlates of bone mass in elderly women. *Journal of Bone and Mineral Research* 1993; 8: 901–908.

108 Frisch RE, Gotz-Welbergen AV, McArthur JW *et al.* Delayed menarche and amenorrhea of college athletes in relation to age of onset of training. *Journal of the American Medical Association* 1981; 246: 1559–1563.

109 Moisan J, Meyer F, Gingras S. A nested case-control study of the correlates of early menarche. *American Journal of Epidemiology* 1990; 132: 953–961.

110 Mustajoki P, Laapio H, Meurman K. Calcium metabolism, physical activity, and stress fractures. *Lancet* 1983; 1: 797.

111 Lanyon LE, Rubin CT, Baust G. Modulation of bone loss during calcium insufficiency by controlled dynamic loading. *Calcified Tissue International* 1986; 38: 209–216.

112 Ferretti JL, Tessaro RD, Audisio EO, Galassi CD. Long-term effects of high or low Ca intakes and of lack of parathyroid function on rat femur biomechanics. *Calcified Tissue International* 1985; 37: 608–612.

113 Specker BL. Evidence for an interaction between calcium intake and physical activity on changes in bone mineral density. *Journal of Bone and Mineral Research* 1996; 11: 1539–1544.

114 Uusirasi K, Sievanen H, Vuori I *et al.* Associations of physical activity and calcium intake with bone mass and size in healthy women at different ages. *Journal of Bone and Mineral Research* 1998; 13: 133–142.

115 Johnston CC, Miller JZ, Slemenda CW *et al.* Calcium supplementation and increases in bone mineral density in children. *New England Journal of Medicine* 1992; 327: 82–87.

116 Lee WTK, Leung SSF, Wang SH *et al.* Double-blind, controlled calcium supplementation and bone mineral accretion in children accustomed to a low-calcium diet. *American Journal of Clinical Nutrition* 1994; 60: 744–750.

117 Matkovic V, Heaney RP. Calcium balance during human growth: evidence for threshold behaviour. *American Journal of Clinical Nutrition* 1992; 55: 992–996.

118 Schwellnus MP, Jordaan G. Does calcium supplementation prevent bone stress injuries? A clinical trial. *International Journal of Sport Nutrition* 1992; 2: 165–174.

119 Myburgh KH, Grobler N, Noakes TD. Factors associated with shin soreness in athletes. *Physician and Sportsmedicine* 1988; 16: 129–134.

120 Gardner LI, Dziados JE, Jones BH *et al.* Prevention of lower extremity stress fractures: a controlled trial of a shock absorbent insole. *American Journal of Public Health* 1988; 78: 1563–1567.

121 Swissa A, Milgrom C, Giladi M *et al.* The effect of pretraining sports activity on the incidence of stress fractures among military recruits. *Clinical Orthopaedics and Related Research* 1989; 245: 256–260.

122 Worthen BM, Yanklowitz BAD. The pathophysiology and treatment of stress fractures in military personnel. *Journal of the American Podiatric Medical Association* 1978; 68: 317–325.

123 Scully TJ, Besterman G. Stress fracture – a preventable training injury. *Military Medicine* 1982; 147: 285–287.

124 Reinker KA, Ozburne S. A comparison of male and female orthopaedic pathology in basic training. *Military Medicine* 1979; August: 532–536.

125 Greaney RB, Gerber RH, Laughlin RL *et al.* Distribution and natural history of stress fractures in U.S. marine recruits. *Radiology* 1983; 146: 339–346.

126 Proztman RR. Physiologic performance of women compared to men. *American Journal of Sports Medicine* 1979; 7: 191–194.

127 Pester S, Smith PC. Stress fractures in the lower extremities of soldiers in basic training. *Orthopaedic Review* 1992; 21: 297–303.

128 Goldberg B, Pecora C. Stress fractures: a risk of increased training in freshmen. *Physician and Sportsmedicine* 1994; 22: 68–78.

129 McBryde AM. Stress fractures in runners. *Clinics in Sports Medicine* 1985; 4: 737–752.

130 Courtenay BG, Bowers DM. Stress fractures: clinical features and investigation. *Medical Journal of Australia* 1990; 153: 155–156.

131 Pecina M, Bojanic I, Dubravcic S. Stress fractures in figure skaters. *American Journal of Sports Medicine* 1990; 18: 277–279.

132 Devas MB, Sweetnam R. Stress fractures of the fibula: a review of fifty cases in athletes. *Journal of Bone and Joint Surgery* 1956; 38B: 818–829.

133 McMahon TA, Greene PR. The influence of track compliance on running. *Journal of Biomechanics* 1979; 12: 893–904.

134 Steele JR, Milburn PD. Effect of different synthetic sport surfaces on ground reaction forces at landing in netball. *International Journal of Sport Biomechanics* 1988; 4: 130–145.

135 Marti B, Vader JP, Minder CE, Abelin T. On the epidemiology of running injuries: the 1984 Bern Grand-Prix study. *American Journal of Sports Medicine* 1988; 16: 285–294.

136 Walter SD, Hart LE, McIntosh JM, Sutton JR. The Ontario cohort study of running-related injuries. *Archives of Internal Medicine* 1989; 149: 2561–2564.

137 Frey C. Footwear and stress fractures. *Clinics in Sports Medicine* 1997; 16: 249–257.

138 Cook SD, Brinker MR, Poche M. Running shoes. *Sports Medicine* 1990; 10: 1–8.

139 Finestone A, Shlamkovitch N, Eldad A, Karp A, Milgrom C. A prospective study of the effect of the appropriateness of foot–shoe fit and training shoe type on the incidence of overuse injuries among infantry recruits. *Military Medicine* 1992; 157: 489–490.

140 Milgrom C, Burr D, Fyhrie D *et al.* The effect of shoe gear on human tibial strains recorded during dynamic loading: a pilot study. *Foot and Ankle International* 1996; 17: 667–671.

141 Cinats J, Reid DC, Haddow JB. A biomechanical evaluation of sorbothane. *Clinical Orthopaedics and Related Research* 1987; 222: 281–288.

142 Voloshin AS, Wosk J. Influence of artificial shock absorbers on human gait. *Clinical Orthopaedics and Related Research* 1981; 160: 52.

143 Milgrom C, Burr DB, Boyd RD *et al.* The effect of a viscoelastic orthotic on the incidence of tibial stress fractures in an animal model. *Foot and Ankle* 1990; 10: 276–279.

144 Milgrom C, Giladi M, Kashtan H *et al.* A prospective study of the effect of a shock-absorbing orthotic device on the incidence of stress fractures in military recruits. *Foot and Ankle* 1985; 6: 101–104.

145 Schwellnus MP, Jordaan G, Noakes TD. Prevention of common overuse injuries by the use of shock absorbing insoles. *American Journal of Sports Medicine* 1990; 18: 636–641.

146 Nigg BM, Herzog W, Read LJ. Effect of viscoelastic shoe insoles on vertical impact forces in heel–toe running. *American Journal of Sports Medicine* 1988; 16: 70–76.

147 Brodsky JW, Kourosh S, Stills M, Mooney V. Objective evaluation of insert material for diabetic and athletic footwear. *Foot and Ankle* 1988; 9: 111–116.

148 Nigg BM. Biomechanics, load analysis and sports injuries in the lower extremities. *Sports Medicine* 1985; 2: 367–379.

[149] Pocock NA, Eisman JA, Hopper J *et al.* Genetic determinants of bone mass in adults. *Journal of Clinical Investigations* 1987; 80: 706–710.

[150] Seeman E, Tsalamandris C, Formica C, Hopper JL, McKay J. Reduced femoral neck bone density in the daughters of women with hip fractures: the role of low peak bone density in the pathogenesis of osteoporosis. *Journal of Bone and Mineral Research* 1994; 9: 739–743.

[151] Soroko SB, Barrett-Connor E, Edelstein SL, Kritz-Silverstein D. Family history of osteoporosis and bone mineral density at the axial skeleton: the Rancho Bernardo study. *Journal of Bone and Mineral Research* 1994; 9: 761–769.

[152] Civitelli R, Ziambaras K. Does Vitamin D receptor gene polymorphism affect bone mineral density and calcium absorption? *Current Opinion in Gastroenterology* 1998; 14: 164–172.

[153] Singer A, Ben-Yehuda O, Bern-Ezra Z, Zaltzman S. Multiple identical stress fractures in monozygotic twins. *Journal of Bone and Joint Surgery* 1990; 72-A: 444–445.

[154] Taimela S, Kujala UM, Osterman K. Intrinsic risk factors and athletic injuries. *Sports Medicine* 1990; 9: 205–215.

Chapter 4

Diagnosis of stress fractures

*D*iagnosis of a stress fracture requires clinical experience, detailed knowledge and precise musculoskeletal examination. In each case, the following three questions have to be answered.
1. Is the pain of bony origin?
2. If so, which bone is involved?
3. At what stage is the injury in the continuum of bone stress (Chapter 1)?
In order to obtain an answer to the three questions, a thorough history, detailed examination and appropriate use of imaging techniques are required. In many cases, diagnosis of stress fracture will be relatively straightforward; in others, especially when the affected bone, for example the femur, may lie deeply, or the pattern of pain, for example navicular, may be nonspecific, diagnosis can present a challenge for the clinician.

History

The history of the stress-fracture patient is typically one of gradual onset of activity-related pain. At first, the pain will usually be described as a mild ache that occurs when a specific amount of exercise is undertaken. If the patient continues to exercise, the pain may well become more severe or occur at an earlier stage of exercise. The pain may increase so that the quality or quantity of the exercise undertaken becomes limited, or, occasionally, all activity is forced to cease. In the early stages, pain will usually cease soon after exercise. However, if exercise is continued and severity of symptoms increases, the pain may persist after exercise. Night pain may occasionally occur.

Although the pain is usually well localized to the site of the fracture, stress fractures of the neck of the femur commonly present with groin pain and occasionally pain referred to the knee, whereas navicular stress fractures usually present with poorly localized foot pain.

It is important to not only obtain a history of the patient's pain and its relation to exercise but to determine the presence of predisposing factors (Chapter 3). A training or activity history is therefore essential. Note should especially be taken of recent changes in activity level such as increased quantity or intensity of training, and of changes made to surface, equipment (mainly shoes) and technique. It may be necessary to obtain training information from the patient's coach or trainer. A full dietary history should be taken, and attention should particularly be paid to the possible presence of an eating disorder. In females, a menstrual history should be taken, including the age at which the woman underwent menarche and her subsequent menstrual status.

A history of a previous similar injury or of any other musculoskeletal injury should be obtained. A review of systems should be obtained in order to assess the patient's general health, medication regimen and personal habits so it can be ensured there are no factors that may influence bone health. It is also important to obtain from the history an understanding of the patient's work and sport commitments. It is especially important to know the level the patient is at, how serious he or she is about his or her sport, and what significant sporting commitments lie ahead for him or her in both the short and medium term.

Physical examination

When physical examination is undertaken, the most obvious feature is localized bony tenderness. This is easier to determine in bones that are relatively superficial, and it may be absent in stress fractures of the shaft or neck of the femur. When palpating the affected areas, particularly regions such as the foot, in which there are a number of bones and joints in a relatively small area, it is important to be anatomically precise. Redness and swelling are occasionally present at the stress-fracture site. There may also be palpable periosteal thickening, especially in a longstanding fracture. Percussion of long bones may result in production of pain at a point distant from the percussion.

Range of joint motion is usually unaffected; the exception is when the stress fracture is close to the joint surface, such as a stress fracture of the neck of the femur. Specific stress fractures may be associated with specific clinical tests. Two examples of the tests are the hang test for stress fractures of the femoral shaft, and hip extension while standing on the contralateral leg, which is used in diagnosis of stress fractures of the pars interarticularis.

Some authors have suggested that the presence of pain when therapeutic ultrasound is applied over the stress-fracture area can be of use in detection of stress fractures.[1–3] However,

Boam *et al.*[4] showed that compared with isotope bone scan, ultrasound sensitivity was only 43% in detection of stress fractures. A high false-positive rate was also evident. Our own experience has not shown this method to be particularly helpful. Similarly, it is reported that application of a vibrating tuning fork to the affected bone and subsequent increase in pain are indicative of a stress fracture. We have also found this method not to be particularly helpful.

When the physical examination is undertaken, the potential intrinsic (Chapter 3) predisposing factors must also be taken into account, and in all stress fractures involving a lower limb, a full biomechanical examination must be performed. Any evidence of leg-length discrepancy, malalignment (especially excessive subtalar pronation), muscle imbalance, muscle weakness, or lack of flexibility should be noted.

Imaging

Imaging has an important supplementary role to play in clinical examination for determining the answers to the three questions outlined at the start of the chapter. In many cases, clinical diagnosis of stress fracture is enough. The classic history of exercise-associated bone pain and typical examination findings of localized bony tenderness are highly correlated with diagnosis of stress fracture. However, if the diagnosis is uncertain, or the case involves the serious or elite athlete who wishes to continue training if at all possible and requires more-specific knowledge of his or her condition, various imaging techniques are available for the clinician. It is essential the clinician use the imaging results as an adjunct to the clinical features, because some of the imaging modalities used for stress fractures are extremely sensitive and may detect subtle abnormalities that are not the cause of the patient's symptoms.

PLAIN RADIOGRAPHY

Plain radiography is widely available and relatively inexpensive. In diagnosis of stress fractures, it has poor sensitivity but high specificity. Unfortunately, in most stress fractures there is no obvious radiographic abnormality. The abnormalities on radiography are unlikely to be seen unless symptoms have been present for at least two to three weeks. In many cases they may not become evident for up to three months, and in a significant percentage of cases they never become abnormal.

In long bones, the first manifestation of a stress fracture is a localized periosteal reaction (Fig. 4.1). Following osteoclastic resorption at the stress-fracture site, a cortical lucency may then become apparent (Fig. 4.2). During healing, the linear stress fracture may undergo resorption around the margin and become an ovoid lucency within a thickened area of cortical hyperostosis. Characteristically, the healing stress fracture will demonstrate thick lamellar periosteal reaction on both the endosteal and periosteal surface confined to a focal area (Fig. 4.3).[5] In an epiphyseal or metaphyseal location, or in a region of mainly cancellous bone (for example calcaneus), focal sclerosis, often band like and representing condensation of trabeculae, is the

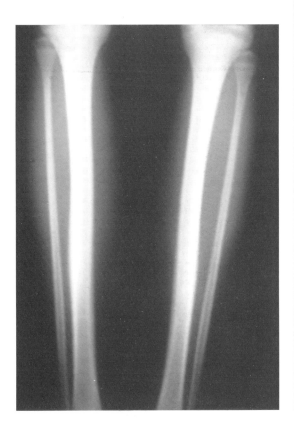

Fig. 4.1
A plain radiograph that shows a periosteal reaction.

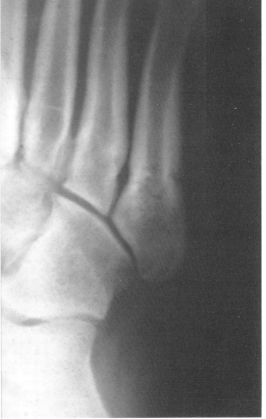

Fig. 4.2
A plain radiograph that shows a fracture line through the cortex.

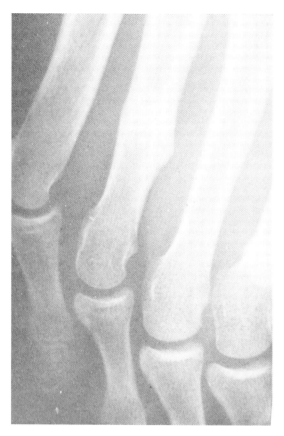

Fig. 4.3
A plain radiograph that shows a healing stress fracture.

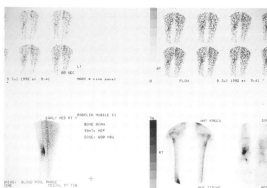

Fig. 4.4
The three phases of an isotope bone scan.

most typical finding, and periostitis is not a prominent feature.[6]

Plain radiography is more likely to demonstrate a stress fracture in long bones such as the tibia, fibula and metatarsal. It should be performed as the first-line investigation in these sites. The plain radiograph is less likely to be helpful in bones such as the femoral shaft, tarsal bones and pars interarticularis.

ISOTOPE BONE SCAN (SCINTIGRAPHY)

If plain radiography demonstrates presence of a stress fracture, there is seldom any need to perform more investigations. However, in cases in which there is a high index of suspicion of

stress fracture, and a negative bone radiograph, the triple-phase bone scan has traditionally been the next line of investigation. The bone scan is highly sensitive but has low specificity. Prather *et al.*[7] stated that the bone scan had a true positive rate of 100%, and false-negative scans are relatively rare.[8,9]

Technetium-99 methylene diphosphonate (Tc-99m) is usually used as the radionuclide substance. Other possibilities include gallium citrate (Ga67) and indium 111-labelled leukocytes.[10] The advantage of Tc-99m is its short (six-hour) half-life, whereby a higher dose with improved resolution is enabled to be administered.[11]

The three phases of an isotope bone scan are shown in Fig. 4.4. In the first phase, flow images are obtained immediately after the tracer has been intravenously injected. These first images are usually taken every two seconds for the first minute and roughly correspond to contrast angiography, although they have much lower spatial and temporal resolution. This first phase of the bone scan evaluates perfusion to bone and soft tissues from the arterial to the venous circulation.

The second phase of the bone scan consists of a static 'blood pool' image taken one minute after the injection and reflects the extent of hyperemia and capillary permeability of bone and soft tissue. Generally, the more acute and severe the injury, the greater the extent of increased perfusion and blood-pool activity.

The third phase of the bone scan is the delayed image taken three to four hours after injection, when approximately 50% of the tracer has concentrated in the bone matrix through the mechanism of chemisorption to the hydroxyapatite crystals. On the three-hour delayed image, the tracer's uptake is proportional to the rate of osteoblastic activity, extraction and efficiency and to the amount of tracer delivered per unit time or blood flow.[12]

In the appropriate clinical setting, scintigraphic diagnosis of a stress fracture is defined as focal increased uptake in the third phase of the bone scan. Inclusion of the bone scan's first and second phases enables the age and severity of stress-induced focal bony lesions to be estimated and helps to differentiate soft-tissue inflammation from bony injury.[13] As the bony lesion heals, the perfusion first returns to normal, and this is followed a few weeks later by normalization of the blood-pool image. Focal increased uptake on the delayed scan resolves last because of ongoing bony remodeling and generally lags well behind disappearance of pain. As healing continues, the intensity of the uptake gradually diminishes over a three- to six-month period following an uncomplicated stress fracture, and a minimal amount of uptake persists for up to ten months,[12] or even longer.

The radionuclide scan may be positive as early as seven hours after bone injury.[14] Matin[15] found that 95% of fractures in patients under sixty-five years of age can be demonstrated on the first day, and in 100% of these patients by three days.

The bone scan is virtually 100% sensitive and much more sensitive than X-ray.[16,17] In several studies, only 10–25% of stress fractures that were bone-scan positive had radiographic evidence of stress fracture.[7,18–21] Radionuclide scanning's sensitivity in demonstrating acute active stress injuries is such that when a scan is

negative, the clinician can be confident that no bony lesion is present.

Bone scan's disadvantage is its lack of specificity in that the fracture itself is not visualized, and it may be difficult to precisely locate the fracture site, especially in the foot. Other nontraumatic lesions such as tumor (especially osteoid osteoma), osteomyelitis, bony infarct, and bony dysplasias can also produce localized increased uptake. It is therefore vitally important to correlate the bone-scan appearance with the clinical features.

In stress fractures, all three phases of the triple-phase bone scan are positive.[13] Other bony abnormalities such as periostitis ('shin splints') are positive on only delayed images (Fig. 4.5),[13,22] whereas some other overuse soft-tissue injuries would be positive only in the angiogram and blood-pool phase, thereby enabling bony pathology and pathology involving soft tissue (Fig. 4.6) to be differentiated.

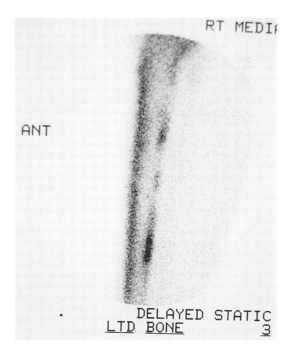

Fig. 4.5
The isotope bone scan appearance of periostitis of the tibia ('shin splints').

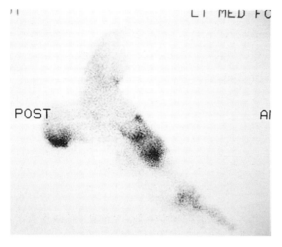

Fig. 4.6
The isotope bone scan appearance of a soft-tissue injury (plantar fasciitis).

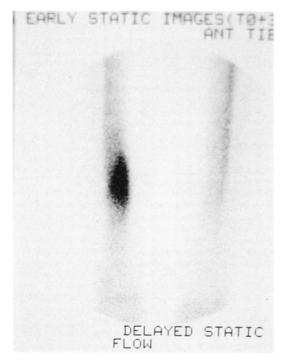

Fig. 4.7
The typical bone scan appearance of a stress fracture.

A stress fracture's characteristic bone-scan appearance is that of a sharply marginated or fusiform area of increased uptake that involves one cortex or occasionally extension of the width of the bone (Fig. 4.7).[23]

The radionuclide scan will detect evolving stress fractures at the stage of accelerated remodeling. At that stage, which may be asymptomatic, the uptake is usually of mild intensity; it progresses to more-intensive and better-defined uptake as microfractures develop.[23] Wilcox *et al.*[24] suggest that the pain associated with a stress fracture may not be present before the radionuclide scan becomes positive.

Increased radionuclide uptake is frequently found in asymptomatic sites (Fig. 4.8).[19,25–27] In athletes, presence of increased tracer uptake at nonpainful sites was originally interpreted to be unrecognized stress fractures.[23,28,29] Other researchers postulated that these may be nonspecific stress changes related to bone remodeling,[13] a false-positive finding,[30] and an uncertain finding.[31] Rosen *et al.*[29] found asymptomatic uptake in 46% of cases and that focal uptake was more common than diffuse uptake.

Matheson and his Vancouver colleagues[19] proposed the concept of bone strain. They noted that because of its sensitivity, radionuclide bone scan was able to demonstrate the adaptive

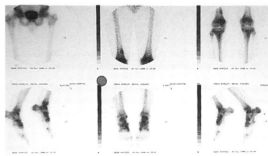

Fig. 4.8
An isotope bone scan that shows multiple areas of increased uptake at asymptomatic sites.

Table 4.1 The continuum of bony changes that occur as a result of overuse

Clinical features	Bone strain	Stress reaction	Stress fracture
Local pain	Nil	Mild to moderate	Mild, moderate, or severe
Local tenderness	Nil	Mild to moderate	Moderate to severe
X-ray appearances	Normal	Normal	May show fracture after 10–14 days
Radioisotopic bone-scan appearance	Increased uptake (mild)	Increased uptake (mild)	Increased uptake (severe)

Source: Adapted and reproduced, with permission, from Brukner PD, Khan KM. Clinical Sports Medicine. *Sydney: McGraw-Hill, 1993: 19 (table 2.5).*

changes in bone at any point in the continuum, from early remodeling to stress fracture. The term 'bone strain' was coined to reflect bone's true dynamic response to stress and to enable interpretation of bone changes along the continuum to be correlated with the wide range of presentations seen in clinical practise. Excessive loading from overuse, abnormal biomechanics, reduced shock absorption, or altered gait produces a mechanical stress that is translated into bone remodeling via piezoelectric stimuli. These factors' relative contribution and the athlete's activity pattern after the onset of remodeling determine the extent of bone strain seen clinically. Pain during activity may indicate small areas of remodeling that have low-intensity uptake on bone scan, and negative X-rays. On the other hand, pain that persists after exercise and during rest may indicate more-extensive remodeling with intensive uptake on scan, and possibly abnormal radiographs.

This concept that a continuum of bone strain exists both clinically and scintigraphically is now widely accepted. It is now clear that bone stress can appear as an area of increased uptake on isotope bone scan before any symptoms occur. It is not clear what percentage of these cases progresses to symptomatic bone stress and ultimately to stress fracture if exercise is continued. It is also not clear what treatment is appropriate in these cases of asymptomatic bone stress. In many athletes and dancers undergoing

Table 4.2 Grading of tibial stress fracture through bone-scan appearance

Grade	Bone-scan appearance
1	Small, ill-defined cortical area of mildly increased activity
2	Better-defined cortical area of moderately increased activity
3	Wide to fusiform cortical–medullary area of highly increased activity
4	Transcortical area of increased activity

hard training, numerous areas of bone stress are shown up on an isotope bone scan. These are indicators of active remodeling and are not necessarily bone at risk for development of stress fracture.

Attempts have been made to classify the bony continuum into 'bone strain' or 'asymptomatic stress reaction' and stress fracture. A summary of these features is set out in Table 4.1.

A scheme for grading bone-scan appearance on the basis of severity has been proposed by Zwas *et al.* (Table 4.2).[21] The researchers found that minimally symptomatic stress fractures were Grade 1 or Grade 2 and that the milder grades' resolution rate was higher with more complete healing. This grading system may help in determining the necessary rest and rehabilitation periods.

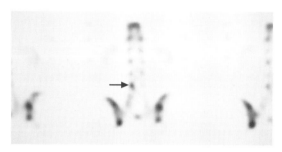

Fig. 4.9
The SPECT appearance of a stress fracture of the pars interarticularis.

Bone scintigraphy's sensitivity can be further increased through use of single photon emission computed tomography (SPECT). Bone SPECT is most helpful in the skeleton's complex areas that have overlapping structures that may obscure pathology, such as the skull, pelvis and spine. It is particularly useful in detection of stress fractures of the pars interarticularis (Fig. 4.9).

COMPUTED TOMOGRAPHY

Computed tomography (CT) is useful for differentiating conditions that have increased uptake on bone scan that may mimic stress fracture. These include osteoid osteoma (Fig. 4.10), osteomyelitis with a Brodie's abscess, and various malignancies.

CT scans are particularly valuable for imaging fractures when imaging may be important in treatment. In particular, CT scanning of the navicular bone (Fig. 4.11) is extremely helpful.[32,33]

CT scanning is also valuable for detecting fracture lines as evidence of stress fracture in long bones (for example metatarsal and tibia) (Fig. 4.12) when plain radiography is normal and isotope bone scan shows increased uptake. CT scanning will enable the clinician to differentiate between a stress fracture that will be visible on CT scan and a stress reaction. Particularly in elite athletes, this may considerably affect

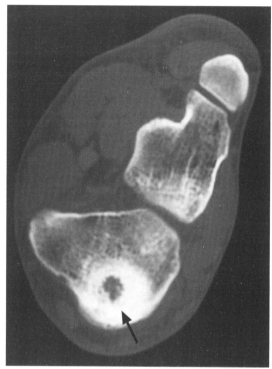

Fig. 4.10
The CT appearance of an osteoid osteoma.

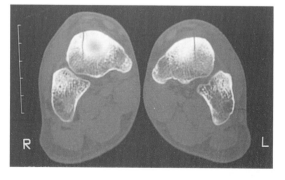

Fig. 4.11
The CT appearance of bilateral stress fractures of the navicular.

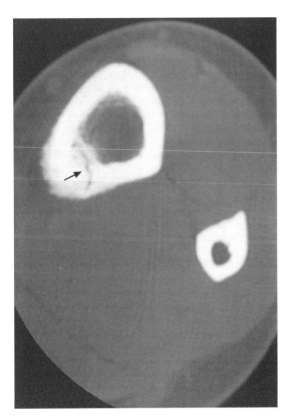

Figure 4.12
The CT appearance of a stress fracture of the tibia.

both their rehabilitation program and their forthcoming competition program.

MAGNETIC RESONANCE IMAGING

For stress fractures, magnetic resonance imaging (MRI) is increasingly being advocated as the investigation of choice. Its sensitivity is similar to that of isotope bone scan, and has the added advantage of excellent anatomic visualization. Unlike bone scan, it will differentiate between stress fracture and tumor, and it will also localize the stress fracture.

Although MRI is performed on a variety of equipment, field strength should be 1.0 to 1.5 T. Total-body scanners have traditionally been used, although the recent advent of dedicated extremity scanners holds the promise of relatively low-cost evaluations. A combination of T1-weighted sequences that optimize anatomic detail and a sequence that depicts bone edema are required for assessment of bone-stress injuries.[34] A variety of edema-sensitive sequences is widely available, and the sequences typically use some form of fat suppression in order to further enhance contrast. Among the widely used edema sequences are short tau inversion recovery (STIR), newer and faster STIR sequences, and fat-suppressed proton density and T2-weighted fast spin echo sequences. Sequences are typically performed in multiple orthogonal planes (for example coronal, sagittal, and axial), and requirements differ, depending on the region of interest.[34]

The earliest evidence of bone stress is appearance of periosteal and/or marrow edema. This shows as an area of reduced signal on T1-weighted sequences and as an area of higher signal (brighter appearance) on T2-weighted sequences (Fig. 4.13). In the absence of clinical symptoms or signs, these areas should be considered to be the equivalent of the areas of increased uptake on bone scan that indicate early bone stress. In the presence of clinical evidence of bone injury and the absence of a fracture line, these appearances should be considered to be evidence of a stress reaction. These areas of edema have an appearance similar to that of bone contusional injuries (bone bruises) as well as to other, less common, conditions such as transient bone marrow edema syndrome, very early osteonecrosis (AVN), osteomyelitis, and infiltrative neoplasm. The findings must be carefully correlated with the clinical symptoms and signs in order to differentiate between the various diagnoses.

On MRI, evidence of a stress fracture is presence of a 'fracture line' that appears as low signal on all sequences. The fracture line is continuous with the cortex and extends into the

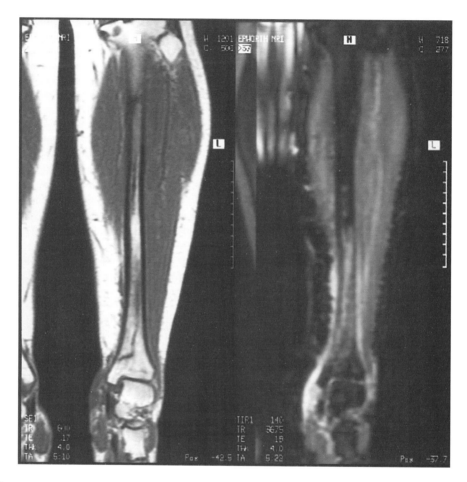

Fig. 4.13
An MRI that shows periosteal and marrow edema in the absence of a fracture line.

intramedullary space oriented perpendicular to the cortex and the major weightbearing trabeculae.[34] The zone of surrounding edema within the medullary space can be very intensive and thereby produce a large amount of abnormal signal loss in the marrow on T1-weighted images. On the T1-weighted images, the fracture line may itself be obscured by the surrounding low-signal edema. Proton density weighted images with fat suppression are excellent for depiction of the fracture line and surrounding edema.[35] On T2-weighted and STIR sequences, the fracture line remains low in signal intensity, and the surrounding marrow edema is seen as an amorphous region of increased signal (Fig. 4.14).[36] Increase in signal on the edema-sensitive sequences becomes less prominent with increasing duration of symptoms. High signal may not be present if the patient is imaged more than four weeks after the onset of symptoms.

In a study by Slocum *et al.*,[37] seven out of ten patients showed resolution of abnormal MRI intensity on STIR images within three months, and nine within six months, of the

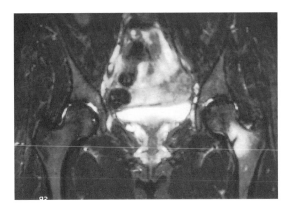

Fig. 4.14

A STIR sequence that shows a fracture line in a zone of marrow edema.

initial diagnosis of stress fracture of the femoral neck.

Arendt *et al.*[38] proposed a grading scheme for MRI appearances of stress fractures, using STIR. This was further modified by Fredericson *et al.*,[39] who used fat-saturated images as the basis of the grading scheme. In this grading system, Grade 1 indicated mild to moderate periosteal edema on T2-weighted images only, with no focal bone marrow abnormality. Grade 2 showed more-severe periosteal edema as well as bone-marrow edema on T2-weighted images only. Grade 3 showed moderate to severe edema of both the periosteum and the marrow on both T1- and T2-weighted images. Grade 4 demonstrated a low-signal fracture line on all sequences, with changes of severe marrow edema on both T1- and T2-weighted images. Grade 4 may also show severe periosteal and moderate muscle edema. Fredericson and colleagues examined runners who had medial shin pain and compared the clinical findings, bone-scan appearances, and MRI appearances. In fourteen out of eighteen symptomatic legs described in the study, MRI findings correlated with the established system for bone-scan grading. The researchers concluded that their Grades 1–4 are equivalent to the bone-scan grading described by Zwas *et al.*,[21] which was mentioned in the previous section.

The comparison of grading of stress fractures between bone scan[21] and MRI[39] is set out in Table 4.3.

Yao *et al.*[40] examined MRI's prognostic value in thirty-five patients who had a suspected stress fracture. An MRI finding of a 'fracture' or 'fatigue' line or of a cortical signal intensity abnormality was predictive of a longer symptomatic period, whereas muscle edema was predictive of a shorter symptomatic period. The researchers did not find that the abovementioned grading system correlated with clinical outcome.

Fredericson *et al.*[39] believed that the MRI more precisely defined the injury's anatomic location and extent. They also identified some clinical symptoms such as pain with daily ambulation, and physical-examination findings, including localized tibial tenderness and pain with direct percussion, that correlated with more-severe grades of bony injuries, in this case in the tibia. The researchers recommended MRI over bone scan for grading of tibial stress lesions and stated that MRI is more accurate for correlating extent of bone involvement with clinical symptoms. Also, MRI bone images involve lack of exposure to ionizing radiation, and imaging time significantly less than that of triple-phase bone scintigraphy. The researchers suggest that periosteal edema represents the tibia's initial response to nontraumatic, repetitive stress, and although the edema can occur in the anterolateral portion of the tibia, it often appears in the same location as most tibial stress fractures: at the posteromedial cortex.

Shin *et al.*[41] compared MRI and isotope bone scan in evaluating the cause of hip pain in endurance athletes. MRI studies were as sensitive as and much more specific than bone scan in determining the cause of hip pain. Isotope bone scan had an accuracy rate of 68% in detecting femoral neck stress fractures and 32% false positives, whereas MRI was 100% accurate. MRI was able to differentiate femoral neck stress fractures from a synovial pit, iliopsoas muscle

Table 4.3 A comparison of stress-fracture appearances, using bone scan and MRI

Bone-scan appearance		MRI appearance
	Grade 1	
Small, ill-defined cortical area of mildly increased activity		Periosteal edema: mild to moderate on T2-weighted images
		Marrow edema: normal on T1- and T2-weighted images
	Grade 2	
Better-defined cortical area of moderately increased activity		Periosteal edema: moderate to severe on T2-weighted images
		Marrow edema on T2-weighted images
	Grade 3	
Wide to fusiform cortical–medullary area of highly increased activity		Periosteal edema: moderate to severe on T2-weighted images
		Marrow edema on T1- and T2-weighted images
	Grade 4	
Transcortical area of increased activity		Periosteal edema: moderate to severe on T2-weighted images
		Marrow edema on T1- and T2-weighted images
		Fracture line clearly visible

(Source: Adapted and reproduced, with permission, from Fredericsson M, Bergman G, Hoffman KL, Dillingham MS. Tibial stress reaction in runners: correlation of clinical symptoms and scintigraphy with a new magnetic resonance imaging grading system. American Journal of Sports Medicine *1995; 23 (4): 472–481.)*

tear, obturator externus tendonitis, avascular necrosis of the femoral head, and a unicameral bone cyst.

BONE SCAN OR MRI?

For stress fractures, the decision to use isotope bone scan or MRI as the investigation of choice is not straightforward. In the vast majority of cases, the combination of clinical presentation, plain radiograph and isotope bone scan is sufficient for a diagnosis of stress fracture. For sensitivity, MRI is comparable to bone scan, and it has the added advantage of visualizing the fracture. However, MRI is considerably more expensive, and the extra cost must be weighed against the added benefit.

Differential diagnosis

Differential diagnosis of stress fracture can be divided into non-bony causes and bony causes. Non-bony causes include muscle or tendon injury, such as muscle strain, hematoma and delayed-onset muscle soreness; and tendon inflammation or degenerative change. Compartment syndrome, especially the lower leg's anterior and deep-posterior compartments, may mimic a stress fracture, because the

SUMMARY

- The typical history of a stress fracture is insidious onset of activity-related pain.
- Localized bony tenderness is the main feature of physical examination.
- Assessment of possible risk factors is an essential part of the history and physical examination.
- A clinical diagnosis of stress fracture is usually sufficient.
- Various imaging techniques are available in order to confirm the diagnosis.
- Plain radiography has low sensitivity but high specificity.
- Isotope bone scan is an extremely sensitive indicator of bone stress but enables neither the fracture to be visualized nor the clinician to determine at what stage of the bone-stress continuum the patient is at.
- MRI is increasingly being used as the investigation of choice.
- MRI is sensitive to the presence of edema, which is an early sign of bone stress.
- In deciding to use bone scan or MRI, the practitioner must weigh up MRI's additional benefits against its increased costs.

syndromes also present with exercise-related pain. Traction periostitis such as that previously termed 'shin splints' or 'medial tibial stress syndrome' may also mimic stress fractures, although the relationship of pain to exercise is different. Bone-scan appearances of both compartment syndrome and periostitis differ from those of stress fracture. Referred pain from the lumbar spine, and vascular pathology such as popliteal artery entrapment, should always be considered in differential diagnosis of exercise-related lower-leg pain.

Bony pathologies that can mimic stress fracture include tumor and infection. Osteoid osteoma is commonly mistaken for a stress fracture because it presents with pain and a discrete focal area of increased uptake on isotope bone scan. Two distinguishing features of osteoid osteoma are presence of night pain and relief of pain with use of aspirin.

References

1 Cole JP, Gossman D. Ultrasonic stimulation of low lumbar nerve roots as a diagnostic procedure: a preliminary report. *Clinical Orthopaedics* 1979; 153: 126.

2 Delacerda FG. A case study: application of ultrasound to determine a stress fracture of the fibula. *Journal of Orthopaedic and Sports Physical Therapy* 1981; 2: 134.

3 Moss A, Mowat AG. Ultrasonic assessment of stress fractures. *British Medical Journal* 1983; 286: 1478.

4 Boam WD, Miser WF, Yuill SC *et al.* Comparison of ultrasound examination with bone scintiscan in the diagnosis of stress fractures. *Journal of American Board of Family Practice* 1996; 9 (6): 414–417.

5 Reeder MT, Dick BH, Atkins JK, Pribis AB, Martinez JM. Stress fractures: current concepts of diagnosis and treatment. *Sports Medicine* 1996; 22 (3): 198–212.

6 Resnick D. Physical injury: concepts and terminology. In: Resnick D, ed. *Diagnosis of Bone and Joint Disorders*. Philadelphia: W. B. Saunders, 1996: 2580–2606.

7 Prather JL, Nusynowitz ML, Snowdy HA *et al.* Scintigraphic findings in stress fractures. *Journal of Bone and Joint Surgery* 1977; 59-A: 869–874.

8 Milgrom C, Chisin R, Giladi M *et al.* Negative bone scans in impending tibial stress fractures: a report of three cases. *American Journal of Sports Medicine* 1984; 12: 488–491.

9 Keene JS, Lash EG. Negative bone scan in a femoral neck stress fracture. *American Journal of Sports Medicine* 1992; 20: 234–236.

10 Monteleone G. Stress fractures in the athlete. *Orthopedic Clinics of North America* 1995; 26 (3): 423–432.

11 Batillas J, Vasilas A, Pizzi WF *et al.* Bone scanning in the detection of occult fractures. *Journal of Trauma* 1981; 21: 564–569.

12 Ammann W, Matheson GO. Radionuclide bone imaging in the detection of stress fractures. *Clinical Journal of Sport Medicine* 1991; 1: 115–122.

13 Rupani HD, Holder LE, Espinola DA, Engin SI. Three-phase radionuclide bone imaging in sports medicine. *Radiology* 1985; 156: 187–196.

14 Rosenthall L, Hill RO, Chuang S. Observation on the use of ^{99m}Tc-phosphate imaging in peripheral bone trauma. *Radiology* 1976; 119: 637–641.

15 Matin P. The appearance of bone scans following fractures, including immediate and long-term studies. *Journal of Nuclear Medicine* 1979; 20: 1227–1231.

16 Taunton JE, Clement DB, Webber D. Lower extremity stress fractures in athletes. *Physician and Sportsmedicine* 1981; 9: 77–86.

17 Saunders AJS, Elsayed TF, Hilson AJW, Maisey MN, Grahame R. Stress lesions of the lower leg and foot. *Clinical Radiology* 1979; 30: 649–651.

18 Milgrom C, Giladi M, Stein M *et al*. Stress fractures in military recruits: a prospective study showing an unusually high incidence. *Journal of Bone and Joint Surgery* 1985; 67-B: 732–735.

19 Matheson GO, Clement DB, McKenzie DC *et al*. Scintigraphic uptake of ^{99m}Tc at non-painful sites in athletes with stress fractures. *Sports Medicine* 1987; 4: 65–75.

20 Clement DB, Ammann W, Taunton JE *et al*. Exercise-induced stress injuries to the femur. *International Journal of Sports Medicine* 1993; 14: 347–352.

21 Zwas ST, Elkanovitch R, Frank G. Interpretation and classification of bone scintigraphic findings in stress fractures. *Journal of Nuclear Medicine* 1987; 28: 452–457.

22 Sterling JC, Edelstein DW, Calvo RD, Webb III R. Stress fractures in the athlete: diagnosis and management. *Sports Medicine* 1992; 14: 336–346.

23 Roub LW, Gumerman LW, Hanley EN *et al*. Bone stress: a radionuclide imaging perspective. *Radiology* 1979; 132: 431–438.

24 Wilcox JR, Moniot AL, Green JP. Bone scanning in the evaluation of exercise-related stress injuries. *Radiology* 1977; 123: 699–703.

25 Greaney RB, Gerber RH, Laughlin RL *et al*. Distribution and natural history of stress fractures in U.S. marine recruits. *Radiology* 1983; 146: 339–346.

26 Lombardo SJ, Benson DW. Stress fractures of the femur in runners. *American Journal of Sports Medicine* 1982; 10: 219–227.

27 Meurman KOA, Elfving S. Stress fracture in soldiers: a multifocal bone disorder. *Radiology* 1980; 134: 483–487.

28 Daffner RH, Martinez S, Gehweiler JA. Stress fractures in runners. *Journal of the American Medical Association* 1982; 247: 1039–1041.

29 Rosen PR, Micheli LJ, Treves S. Early scintigraphic diagnosis of bone stress and fractures in athletic adolescents. *Pediatrics* 1982; 70: 11–15.

30 Geslien GE, Thrawl JH, Espinosa JL, Older RA. Early detection of stress fractures using ^{99m}Tc-polyphosphate. *Radiology* 1976; 121: 683–687.

31 Butler JE, Brown SL, McConnell BG. Subtrochanteric stress fractures in runners. *American Journal of Sports Medicine* 1982; 10: 228–232.

32 Khan KM, Fuller PJ, Brukner PD, Kearney C, Burry HC. Outcome of conservative and surgical management of navicular stress fracture in athletes. *American Journal of Sports Medicine* 1992; 20: 657–666.

33 Kiss ZA, Khan KM, Fuller PJ. Stress fractures of the tarsal navicular bone: CT findings in 55 cases. *American Journal of Roentgenology* 1993; 160: 111–115.

34 Deutsch AL, Coel MN, Mink JH. Imaging of stress injuries to bone: radiography, scintigraphy and MR imaging. *Clinics in Sports Medicine* 1997; 16 (2): 275–290.

35 Kapelov SR, Teresi LM, Bradley WG *et al*. Bone contusions of the knee: increased lesion detection with fast spin echo MR imaging with spectroscopic fat saturation. *Radiology* 1993; 189: 901.

36 Meyers SP, Wiener SN. Magnetic resonance imaging features of fractures using the short tau inversion (STIR) sequence: correlation with radiographic findings. *Skeletal Radiology* 1991; 20: 4999–5007.

37 Slocum KA, Gorman JD, Puckett ML, Jones SB. Resolution of abnormal MR signal intensity in patients with stress fractures of the femoral neck. *American Journal of Roentgenology* 1997; 168 (5): 1295–1299.

38 Arendt L, Griffiths HJ, Galloway HR *et al*. The MR spectrum of stress injury to bone and its clinical relevance. *American Journal of Sports Medicine* 1997; (In press.).

39 Fredericsson M, Bergman G, Hoffman KL, Dillingham MS. Tibial stress reaction in runners: correlation of clinical symptoms and scintigraphy with a new magnetic resonance imaging grading system. *American Journal of Sports Medicine* 1995; 23 (4): 472–481.

40 Yao L, Johnson C, Gentili A, Lee JK, Seeger LL. Stress injuries of bone – analysis of MR staging criteria. *Academic Radiology* 1998; 5 (1): 34–40.

41 Shin AY, Morin WD, Gorman JD, Jones SB, Lapinsky AS. The superiority of magnetic resonance imaging in differentiating the cause of hip pain in endurance athletes. *American Journal of Sports Medicine* 1996; 24 (2): 168–176.

Chapter 5

Treatment of stress fractures

*F*or athletes, the actual time from when a stress fracture is diagnosed to when they can fully return to their sport depends on a number of factors, including the fracture site, the symptoms, duration and the lesion's severity (the stage in the bone-strain continuum).

Most stress fractures for which there is a relatively brief history of symptoms will heal without complication or delay, and return to sport will be permitted within the four- to eight-week range. However, a group of stress fractures exists for which additional treatment and special consideration are required. These stress fractures are listed later in the summary on page 103.

Although many subtleties are involved in stress-fracture management, the main treatment is modified activity. During the modified-activity phase, a number of important issues are attended to, including modification of risk factors, maintenance of muscular strength and fitness, management of pain, investigation of bone health, and prescription of orthotic devices. Stress-fracture care is divided into two phases: Phase 1, early treatment using modified activity, and Phase 2, the period from reintroduction of physical activity to full return to sport.

Phase 1

MANAGEMENT OF PAIN

Although pain is seldom severe, it can be a problem, even when normal walking is undertaken. Mild analgesics or nonsteroidal anti-inflammatories (NSAIDs) can be used, as well as physical-therapy modalities (for example ice, and interferential electrical stimulation). In some cases in which daily-living activities are painful, it may be necessary for the stress-fracture patient to be non-weightbearing or partially weightbearing on crutches for a period of up to seven to ten days. In most cases this is not necessary, and mere avoidance of the aggravating activity will be sufficient.

MUSCULAR STRENGTH AND ENDURANCE

In Chapter 1 we discussed skeletal muscle's important function in providing shock absorption in order to reduce the magnitude of the load delivered to the axial skeleton. In endurance sports, even low levels of muscular fatigue can possibly affect the total-impact load to bone, particularly in the athlete's lower extremity. In the clinical setting, decrements in muscular strength and endurance may be undetectable whether testing is performed manually or using a machine such as an isokinetic dynamometer. Muscular strength as measured by the torque generated by a single contraction against resistance is a function of stored adenosine triphosphate (ATP) and phosphocreatine (PCr) as well as of neural factors. A more important measure is the muscle's fatiguability, which is a function of additional factors, including substrate supply and use.

Because muscular strength and endurance are so important and subtle abnormalities are nevertheless difficult to detect clinically, all athletes who have a stress fracture of the lower extremity should receive a specific program of muscle-strengthening exercises for muscle groups surrounding the joints above and below the fracture line. Muscle-strengthening programs are usually prescribed for a period of six weeks and begin immediately after the stress fracture has been diagnosed.

MAINTENANCE OF FITNESS

Fitness maintenance during periods of forced inactivity as a result of injury is a major concern for coaches and athletes. Inactivity has marked effects on the cardiovascular system as well as on skeletal muscle's metabolic and morphologic characteristics. Reduction in various fitness parameters has been reported after athletes have had relatively brief periods of inactivity. Decrements in maximal stroke volume, cardiac output, and maximal oxygen uptake of approximately 25% have been reported after athletes have had twenty days of bed rest.[1] Other studies have shown a 14% to 16% decline in maximal oxygen uptake when training has been ceased for six weeks.[2,3]

The effect of rest on performance varies from one athlete to another and depends on the specific sport. It is important that the athlete who has a stress fracture be able to maintain strength and cardiovascular fitness during Phase 1. It should be emphasized to the athlete that during Phase 1, the rehabilitation program is designed to neither maintain nor improve the patient's fitness but to enable the damaged bone to have time to heal and gradually develop or regain full strength. Fitness should be maintained in ways whereby loading of the bone is avoided.

Nonloading activities through which fitness is maintained are the ones in which as many large-muscle groups as possible are used without loading of the bone. Recruitment of many large muscles results in high oxygen uptake, and in substituting a nonloading activity for the athlete's sport, the goal is to place an equal or greater demand on the cardiopulmonary system in order to supply large quantities of oxygen to the working muscles. The most common fitness-maintenance methods are cycling, swimming, water running, rowing, and stairmaster. For muscular strength, upper- and lower-body weight programs can usually be prescribed without promoting risk. As much as possible, these workouts should mimic the athlete's normal training program in both duration and intensity.

Deep-water running (DWR), which involves immersion up to the neck and use of a vest as a flotation device, is particularly attractive for runners because it closely simulates their sport. In training studies in which DWR and land running were compared, no significant differences in maximal oxygen uptake,[4-6] anaerobic threshold, running economy,[6] leg strength,[4] and two-mile performance[5] were reported after land training versus DWR training was undertaken for four to eight weeks. Avellini et al.[7] reported similar improvements in land maximal oxygen uptake after a twelve-week DWR program was compared to a land cycling ergometer program. In another study,[8] it was shown that competitive runners are able to achieve training intensities similar to those of land running for water-immersion running with or without a flotation vest. However, recreational runners failed to replicate land-training pace.

DWR's effectiveness is dependent on simulation of land-based running style and workouts in the water. However, DWR is not identical to land running, and some important differences must be taken into account when a DWR program is being set. Because of the water environment's viscosity friction and DWR's non-weightbearing nature, this form of running is mechanically different from land running. In DWR, stride frequency has been reported to be 60% to 65% that of land values.[9] Although heart rate can be used for monitoring exercise intensity in DWR sessions, it is important to note that water immersion results in a cephalad shift in blood volume, which during water-immersion exercise results in increase in stroke volume[10] and decline in maximal heart rate.[9–11] The effect of water immersion on heart rate has been reported to be approximately ten to thirteen beats per minute lower when exercising at high work loads but similar to land values at lower intensities of exercise.[12]

It is possible to maintain fitness in even elite athletes. Frangolias *et al.*[13] reported the case of an elite middle-distance runner who sustained a Jones' fracture (see Chapter 10) of the right foot for which a lengthy (ten- to twelve-week) period of non-weightbearing cast immobilization was required. Only limited activity was allowed during the first three weeks after injury, because of discomfort. A more structured program that consisted of a six-day training and one-day rest schedule was initiated in week 4 (Table 5.1). Although treadmill VO_2max and ventilatory threshold showed small decreases, progressive improvement was noted in both parameters at twenty-three and thirty weeks post-injury. Ten-kilometer-race performance at thirty-one weeks post-injury was six seconds faster than the athlete's pre-injury time.

Although VO_2max and muscular strength have been shown to be maintained through alternative activities, specific metabolic and neuromuscular adaptatations that affect skill are not easily duplicated. For this reason, isolated skill-related activities are resumed as early as possible during Phase 1. In most cases, it is possible for the athlete to maintain specific-sport skills. In ball sports, these can involve the athlete in activities either seated or standing still. This active-rest approach also greatly assists the athlete psychologically.

MODIFICATION OF RISK FACTORS

As is the case with any overuse injury, it is not enough to merely treat the stress fracture itself. Stress fractures are the result of subtle, incremental overload. Making subtle adjustments to the modifiable factors that contribute to the total load is an essential component of management of an athlete who has a stress fracture. By obtaining a thorough history, the practitioner identifies the factors that have

Table 5.1 A weekly water-running training regimen

Day	Training regimen
1	Interval training, and simulated-mile repeats: 4×5 minutes to 6×5 minutes, including 1 minute's rest; heart rate = 175–180 beats per minute
2	Low-intensity run: 30–45 minutes; heart rate = 130–150 beats per minute
3	Interval training: hard intervals – 6×3 minutes, including 1 minute's rest; heart rate = 175–180 beats per minute
4	Low-intensity run, as for day 2
5	Interval training: short – $5–15 \times 2$ minutes or $5–15 \times 1$ minute, including 30 seconds' rest; heart rate = 175–180 beats per minute
6	Long, steady-state run: 40–90 minutes; heart rate = 145–165 beats per minute
7	Rest day (or low-intensity run)

(Source: Adapted and reproduced, with permission, from Frangolias DD et al. Maintenance of aerobic capacity during recovery from right Jones' fracture. (Case report). Clinical Journal of Sport Medicine 1997; 7 (1): 54–58.)

contributed to the injury and the ones that can be modified so that the risk of injury recurrence is reduced. The fact that stress fractures have a high recurrence rate is an indication that this part of the management program is often neglected.

In Chapter 3, the risk factors for stress-fracture development were discussed at length. The most common precipitating factors are probably training errors. It is therefore important that these be identified and discussed with the athlete and his or her coach when appropriate. Training errors include a sudden or rapid increase in training volume or intensity, at least at a rate greater than that required for bone's adequate adaptation. Coaches have to be reminded that training regimens for athletes must be individualized. What may be appropriate for some team members may be excessive for others.

Another important contributing factor may be inadequate equipment, especially running shoes. These shoes may be inappropriate for the athlete's foot type, have general inadequate support or be worn out. Shoes should be replaced approximately every 500 kilometers. It is more important that shoes be replaced frequently than that the most expensive pair available be purchased.

It is also believed that intrinsic biomechanic abnormalities are a contributing factor in development of overuse injuries in general and of stress fractures in particular. Varus alignment, and either excessively supinated or excessively pronated feet may contribute to stress-fracture development. Excessively supinated feet (pes cavus) generally give limited shock absorption and require footwear that compensates for this. Excessively pronated feet increase the amount of tibial torsion during gait and require appropriate footwear or custom-made foot orthoses in order to control the excessive amount of pronation.

Management of the amenorrheic female athlete who has a stress fracture is controversial, and it is suggested that each case be treated individually. It may be possible to persuade the athlete to reduce the amount and intensity of her activity and/or to increase her body fat, both of which changes may enable her menses to resume their normal pattern. If the athlete is unwilling or unable to follow this course, the possibility of hormonal supplementation should be discussed. The hormones are usually taken in the form of one of the low-dose oral contraceptive pills (OCPs). However, there has traditionally been considerable resistance by serious athletes to taking the OC pill on the grounds they could cause weight gain. The role of bone-density measurement in these patients remains unclear. In bone-density measurement, the patient's bone density is compared to the 'average', but it is known that bone density is increased in females involved in weightbearing exercise. Bone-density measurement can be useful in this group, both for providing a baseline measurement before treatment is commenced and as an additional factor (if the measurement is reduced) in persuading the athlete to commence treatment.

If after assessment of the athlete's dietary intake there is evidence of inadequate overall caloric or calcium intake, the clinician should give dietary advice or the athlete should be referred to a dietitian. Athletes who have a stress fracture should consume 1500 milligrams of calcium and 400 to 800 international units of Vitamin D per day.

It is important that these risk factors be corrected by the time the athlete resumes training.

Phase 2

When normal day-to-day ambulation is pain free, resumption of the impact-loading activities begins. The rate of activity resumption should be modified according to symptoms and physical findings. For lower-limb stress fractures for which running is the aggravating activity, a program is recommended that first involves brisk walking increased by five to ten minutes per day up to a length of forty-five minutes. Although pain should not accompany activity resumption, it is not uncommon for the patient to have some discomfort at the stress-fracture site. If bony pain occurs, activity should be ceased for one to two days. If normal ambulation is pain free, the activity should be resumed at the volume and pace below the level at which the pain occurred. The patient should be clinically reassessed at fortnightly intervals, in order to assess the training program's progress and any symptoms related to the stress fracture.

Once forty-five minutes of continuous brisk walking is achieved without pain, slow jogging can begin for a period of five minutes within the walk. Assuming that this increase in activity does not reproduce the patient's symptoms, the amount of jogging can be increased by five minutes per session on either a daily or an every-other-day basis to a total of forty-five minutes at slow-jogging pace. This period of time is necessary in order to load the bone slowly and to ensure that adequate healing has occurred. Once the goal of forty-five minutes is achieved, pace can be increased: half-pace at first, gradually increased to full-pace striding. Once full sprinting is achieved pain free, functional activities such as hopping, skipping, jumping, twisting, and turning can be introduced gradually. It is important that this process be a

graduated one, and it is important to err on the side of caution, not to try to return too quickly.

A typical program for resuming activity for an uncomplicated lower-limb stress fracture after a period of initial rest and daily-living activities is set out in Table 5.2.

This pattern of activity reintroduction can be followed for other sports. For aerobics classes, for example, reintroduction of aerobic floor exercises should begin at two minutes per session, and the remaining eighteen minutes of 'cardio' should be spent on the exercise bike. This ratio is gradually increased until the patient is back to full-time floor exercise.

It is not infrequent that the patient experiences pain at some point during activity reintroduction. This is by no means an indication of a return of the stress fracture. In each instance, the activity should be discontinued, there should be several days of modified rest, and training should resume at a level lower than that at which the pain occurred. If the clinician places the patient on an accelerated program for activity reintroduction, monitoring periods should be adjusted accordingly and in some cases be weekly. Progress should be monitored clinically by way of presence or absence of symptoms, and local signs. It is not necessary to monitor progress by

Table 5.2 An activity program after an uncomplicated lower-limb stress fracture following a period of rest and activities of daily living (ADL)

	Day 1	Day 2	Day 3	Day 4	Day 5	Day 6	Day 7
				Number of minutes			
Week 1	Walk 15.	Walk 20.	Walk 25.	Walk 30.	Walk 35.	Walk 40.	Walk 45.
Week 2	Walk 20. Jog 5. Walk 20.	Walk 15. Jog 10. Walk 15.	Walk 15. Jog 15. Walk 15.	Walk 10. Jog 20. Walk 10.	Walk 10. Jog 25. Walk 10.	Walk 5. Jog 30. Walk 5.	Walk 5. Jog 35. Walk 5.
Week 3	Walk 5. Jog 40.	Jog 45.	Jog 35. Stride 10.	Jog 30. Stride 15.	Jog 30. Stride 20.	Jog 35. Sprint 10.	Jog 30. Sprint 15.
Week 4	Add functional activities.			Gradually increase all week.			
Week 5				Resume full training.			

way of radiography, scintigraphy, CT or MRI, because radiologic healing often lags behind clinical healing.

When training resumes, it is important that recovery time be adequate after hard sessions or hard weeks of training. This need can be accommodated by developing microcycles and macrocycles. Alternating hard and easy training sessions is a microcycle adjustment, but graduating the volume of work or alternating harder and easier sessions can also be undertaken either weekly or monthly. In view of the history of stress fracture, it is advisable that some form of cross-training, for example swimming and cycling for a runner, be introduced in order to reduce the stress on the previously injured area and to reduce the likelihood of a recurrence.

BRACING

Rest from the aggravating activity has traditionally been the cornerstone of stress-fracture treatment. However, clinicians and the athletes themselves are continually looking for a way to accelerate the healing process and reduce the time for returning to sport. A number of methods have been used.

In a number of studies, use of a long pneumatic leg brace (Aircast) has resulted in a positive effect on time for returning to play after a tibial stress fracture has occurred. Dickson and Kichline[14] reported on thirteen consecutive female athletes for whom sixteen tibial or fibular stress fractures were diagnosed. All the fractures were treated with a pneumatic leg brace, and the athletes were able to return to their sport immediately, without disabling symptoms. However, the study involved a number of problems. When the patients who did not have confirmed stress fractures and the fibular stress fractures were excluded from the group, seven tibial stress fractures remained. The average time from onset of symptoms to diagnosis was six weeks, and the average time to

disappearance of all symptoms was 3.4 weeks, although all athletes immediately resumed their sport.

Whitelaw et al.[15] reported on twenty tibial stress fractures that occurred in seventeen competitive athletes. The diagnosis was made by way of either positive bone scan or positive radiograph. All the patients were fitted with a pneumatic leg brace. Activity resumption occurred after an average 3.7 weeks, and return to full, unrestricted activity occurred after an average 5.3 weeks. The researchers claimed that this result represented a significant improvement when compared with traditional treatment. They considered the traditional time of return to full activity to be twelve weeks, based on Matheson et al.,[16] although in our clinical experience, athletes return to full activity at an average of eight weeks. Neither of these two studies, however, had a control group.

Swenson et al.[17] undertook a prospective controlled study of pneumatic-brace use in treatment of tibial stress fractures. Patients were randomly assigned to the traditional ($n = 8$) or brace ($n = 10$) group. The median time from initiation of treatment to the beginning of light activity was seven days for the brace group and twenty-one days for the traditional group. The brace group became pain free on hopping at a median fourteen days after initiation of treatment, compared with a median forty-five days for the traditional group. The time from initiation of treatment to completion of a standard functional-progression program was twenty-one days, compared with seventy-seven days for the traditional group.

On the basis of the lastmentioned study, patients who have a tibial stress fracture may well benefit from being placed in a long (40 centimeter) pneumatic leg brace at the time of diagnosis. It is important it be remembered that accelerated healing of the stress fractures has not been shown in these studies – only accelerated activity resumption. More studies have to be done in this area.

Swenson and colleagues propose that the pneumatic leg brace shifts a portion of the weightbearing load from the tibia to the soft tissue and that this results in less impact loading when walking, hopping, and running are undertaken. They also suggest that the brace facilitates healing at the fracture site by acting to compress the soft tissue; this thereby increases the intravascular hydrostatic pressure and results in a shifting of the fluid and electrolytes from the capillary space to the interstitial space. The piezoelectric effect is theoretically enhanced, and osteoblastic bone formation is enhanced.

Although no studies have been conducted on the pneumatic leg brace's effect on other lower-limb stress fractures, it is reasonable to assume that the brace might have a positive effect on healing of fractures at other sites.

ELECTRICAL STIMULATION

Various methods of electrical stimulation have all been shown to have a positive effect on healing of nonunited traumatic fractures. The methods include pulsed electromagnetic fields,[17–25] direct electric current,[26–29] and capacitively coupled electric field.[27,30–34] No studies have been conducted of this treatment's efficacy in nonunion of stress fractures, and only one nonblinded, uncontrolled study has been conducted of its effect on time for returning to sport with reference to stress fractures in athletes.

Benazzo *et al.*[35] reported the results of a study on treatment of stress fractures in athletes by way of capacitive coupling: a bone healing-stimulation method in which bone formation is promoted by way of application of alternating current in the form of a sinusoidal wave. Twenty-two out of twenty-five stress fractures were healed, and two more showed improvement. Most of the fractures were stress fractures of the navicular and fifth metatarsal, which are prone to delayed union or nonunion. More double-blinded controlled studies are required in order to determine this treatment's efficacy in management of both the acute stress fracture and non-union of stress fractures.

SURGERY

Surgery is virtually never required in management of the routine stress fracture. However, it may be required in the case of displaced stress fracture (for example the neck of the femur) or established non-union (for example the anterior cortex of the tibia). Specific fractures for which surgery may be required are discussed in the chapters in which the regions are discussed.

STRESS FRACTURES FOR WHICH SPECIFIC TREATMENT IS REQUIRED

SUMMARY

Although most stress fractures will heal without complications within a relatively short timeframe, for a number of stress fractures the tendency exists for the athlete to develop complications, such as delayed union or nonunion, for which specific additional treatment is required. These stress fractures are
- the neck of the femur
- the pars interarticularis
- the patella
- the anterior cortex, midshaft tibia
- the medial malleolus
- the talus
- the navicular
- the fifth metatarsal
- the second metatarsal (base)
- the sesamoid.

Specific management for these stress fractures is described in the chapter for each region.

References

1 Saltin B, Blomqvist G, Mitchell JH *et al.* Response to submaximal and maximal exercise after bed rest and training. *Circulation* 1968; 38 (Suppl 7).

2 Pedersen PK, Jorgensen K. Maximal oxygen uptake in young women with training, inactivity and retraining. *Medicine Science in Sports and Exercise* 1978; 10: 223–237.

3 Coyle EF, Martin WH, Sinacore DR. Time course of loss of adaptations after stopping prolonged intense endurance training. *Journal of Applied Physiology* 1984; 57: 1857–1864.

4 Hertler L, Provost-Craig M, Sestili D. Water running and the maintenance of maximum oxygen consumption and leg strength in runners. (Abstract). *Medicine and Science in Sports and Exercise* 1992; 24: S23.

5 Eyestone ED, Fellingham G, George J. Effect of water running and cycling on maximum oxygen consumption and 2 mile run performance. *American Journal of Sports Medicine* 1993; 21: 41–44.

6 Wilber RL, Moffatt RJ, Scott BE. Influence of water-run training on running performance. (Abstract). *Medicine and Science in Sports and Exercise* 1994; 26: S4.

7 Avellini BA, Shapiro Y, Pandolf KB. Cardiorespiratory physical training in water and on land. *European Journal of Applied Physiology* 1983; 50: 255–263.

8 Gehring MM, Keller BA, Brehm BA. Water running with and without a flotation vest in competitive and recreational runners. *Medicine and Science in Sports and Exercise* 1997; 29 (10): 1374–1378.

9 Frangolias DD, Rhodes EC. Maximal and ventilatory threshold responses to treadmill and water immersion running. *Medicine and Science in Sports and Exercise* 1995; 27 (7): 1007–1013.

10 Christie JL, Shelddahl LM, Tristani FE *et al.* Cardiovascular regulation during head-out water immersion exercise. *Journal of Applied Physiology* 1990; 69: 657–664.

11 Butts NK, Tucker M, Greening C. Physiological responses to maximal treadmill and deep water running in men and women. *American Journal of Sports Medicine* 1991; 19: 612–614.

12 Frangolias DD, Rhodes EC, Belcastro AN *et al.* Comparison of metabolic responses of prolonged work at Tvent during treadmill and water immersion running. (Abstract). *Medicine and Science in Sports and Exercise* 1994; 26: S10.

13 Frangolias DD, Taunton JE, Rhodes EC *et al.* Maintenance of aerobic capacity during recovery from right Jones' fracture. (Case report). *Clinical Journal of Sport Medicine* 1997; 7 (1): 54–58.

14 Dickson TB, Kichline PD. Functional management of stress fractures in female athletes using a pneumatic leg brace. *American Journal of Sports Medicine* 1987; 15: 86–89.

15 Whitelaw GP, Wetzler MJ, Levy AS, Segal D, Bissonett K. A pneumatic leg brace for the treatment of tibial stress fractures. *Clinical Orthopedics Related Research* 1991; 270: 302–305.

16 Matheson GO, Clement DB, McKenzie DC *et al.* Stress fractures in athletes: a study of 320 cases. *American Journal of Sports Medicine* 1987; 15: 46–58.

17 Swenson EJ, DeHaven KE, Sebastienelli WJ *et al.* The effect of a pneumatic leg brace on return to play in athletes with tibial stress fractures. *American Journal of Sports Medicine* 1997; 25 (3): 322–328.

18 Bassett CAL, Pawluk RJ, Becker RO. Augmentation of bone repair by inductively coupled electromagnetic fields. *Science* 1974; 184: 575–577.

19 Bassett CAL, Mitchell SN, Norton L, Pilla A. A non-operative salvage of surgically-resistant pseudarthroses and non-unions by pulsating electromagnetic fields: a preliminary report. *Clinical Orthopaedics* 1977; 124: 128.

20 Bassett CAL, Mitchell SN, Norton L. Repair of non-union by pulsing electromagnetic fields. *Acta Orthopedica Belge* 1978; 44: 706–724.

21 Bassett CAL, Mitchell SN, Gaston SR. Treatment of ununited tibial diaphyseal fractures with pulsing electromagnetic fields. *Journal of Bone and Joint Surgery* 1981; 63-A: 511–523.

22 Barker AT, Dixon RA, Sharrard WJ, Sutcliffe ML. Pulsed magnetic field therapy for tibial non-union: interim results of a double-blind trial. *Lancet* 1984; 1: 994–996.

23 O'Connor BT. Pulsed magnetic field therapy for tibial non-union. *Lancet* 1984; 2: 171–172.

24 De Haas WG, Beaupre A, Cameron H, English E. The Canadian experience with pulsed magnetic fields in the treatment of ununited tibial stress fractures. *Clinical Orthopedics* 1986; 208: 55–58.

25 Sharrard WJW. A double-blind trial of pulsed electromagnetic fields for delayed union of tibial fractures. *Journal of Bone and Joint Surgery* 1990; 72-B (3):347–355.

26 Brighton CT, Black J, Friedenberg ZB *et al.* A multicenter study of the treatment of non-union with constant direct current. *Journal of Bone and Joint Surgery* 1981; 63-A: 2–13.

27 Brighton CT, Shaman P, Heppenstall RB *et al.* Tibial nonunion treated with direct current, capacitive coupling, or bone graft. *Clinical Orthopaedics* 1995; 321: 223–234.

28 Esterhai JL, Brighton CT, Heppenstall RB, Alavi A, Desai AG. Detection of synovial pseudarthrosis by 99mTc

scintigraphy: application to treatment of traumatic non-union with constant direct current. *Clinical Orthopaedics* 1981; 161: 15–23.

29 Parnell EJ, Simons RB. The effect of electrical stimulation in the treatment of non-union of the tibia. *Journal of Bone and Joint Surgery* 1991; 73-B: S178.

30 Brighton CT, Pollock SR. Treatment of non-union of the tibia with a capacitively coupled electric field. *Journal of Traumatology* 1984; 24: 153.

31 Brighton CT, Pollock SR. Treatment of recalcitrant nonunion with a capacitively coupled electric field: a preliminary report. *Journal of Bone and Joint Surgery* 1985; 67-A: 577–585.

32 Brand PW, Beach RB, Thompson DE. Relative tension and potential excursion of muscles in the forearm and hand. *Journal of Hand Surgery* 1981; 3: 209–219.

33 Brighton CT, McCluskey WP. The early response of bone cells in culture to a capacitively coupled electric field. *Trans Biolectric Repair and Growth Society* 1983; 3: 10.

34 Scott G, King JB. A prospective, double blind trial of electrical capacitive coupling in the treatment of non-union of long bones. *Journal of Bone and Joint Surgery* 1994; 76-A (6): 820–826.

35 Benazzo F, Mosconi M, Beccarisi G, Galli U. Use of capacitive coupled electric fields in stress fractures in athletes. *Clinical Orthopaedics and Related Research* 1995; 310: 145–149.

Chapter 6

Stress fractures of the upper limb

*A*lthough stress fractures of the upper limb are much less common than stress fractures of the lower limb, they have been described with reference to sports dominated by the upper limbs, such as tennis, swimming, and throwing activities. These stress fractures have been reported in individual case reports, but no large series have been published in the literature.

The clavicle

Although stress fractures of the clavicle have been described as being a late complication following radical neck dissection,[1,2] only two cases of clavicular stress fracture in athletes have been reported.[3,4]

One case was that of a 25-year-old, male, right-handed, elite-javelin thrower;[3] the other was that of a collegiate springboard diver.[4] The two athletes presented with insidious onset of pain over the clavicle, and local tenderness. The pain was maximal when the shoulder was abducted above the horizontal plane. Radiographs showed periosteal reaction in both cases, and the diagnosis was confirmed by way of isotope bone scan in one case and plain tomography in the other. Both athletes returned to full activity after eight weeks. With reference to the javelin thrower, the researchers postulated that repeated stress from contraction of the clavicular portions of the deltoid and pectoralis major muscles contributed to development of the fracture. With reference to the diver, it was believed that the position on water entry, whereby the fingers and wrists were extended, the forearms were pronated and the hands were overlapping, may have transmitted impact stress from the hands to the clavicle.

The scapula

Stress fractures of the scapula are also rare. Reports exist of scapula body stress fracture related to occupation. Three stress fractures in truck drivers[5-7] and one stress fracture in an overhead worker who worked on a car-assembly line[8] have been reported in the literature. With reference to athletes, scapular stress fractures have been reported in a gymnast[9] and a jogger who was using hand-held weights.[10] A stress fracture of the base of the acromial process has been reported in a professional football player,[11] and a coracoid-process stress fracture has been reported in a trap shooter.[12]

Veluvolu *et al.*[10] report the case of a thirty-year-old man who had been jogging with hand-held weights for about eight weeks. The man complained he had had pain in the right shoulder for two weeks. An isotope bone scan showed a linear band of increased uptake in the superomedial portion of the right scapula superior to the spinous process. Later radiographs showed a fracture through the region. The researchers state that the likely cause was overuse of muscle fibers of the supraspinatus in stabilizing the humeral head while the man was jogging with weights.

Ward *et al.*[11] describe a 28-year-old male offensive lineman who had no history of significant trauma but developed pain in the shoulder during a football game. He had not noticed pain before the game but had been lifting weights in an intensive prescribed program. Physical examination revealed point tenderness over the acromion, and pressure applied to the tip of the acromion caused pain at the base of the acromial arch. Anteroposterior, lateral, West Point and modified oblique-view radiographs showed an incomplete transverse radiolucent line in an area of sclerotic bone at the underside of the acromion near its origin from the scapula spine. The fracture was best seen by way of tomography. A technetium bone scan revealed increased activity in the region. The player's weightlifting and football activities were discontinued for six weeks. After that, he gradually resumed weightlifting and contact-sport activities and was playing competitive football within two months with neither pain nor tenderness. Two months later, follow-up radiographs showed callus in the fracture area. The researchers believe that the intense weightlifting program contributed to development of the stress fracture.

Stress fracture of the coracoid process has been described in association with trap shooting.[12] A 27-year-old female professional trap shooter regularly shot trap at the rate of 200 to 1000 rounds per week. She complained of aching in the shoulder at the point at which the butt of the rifle rests. Physical examination showed that the patient had point tenderness directly over the coracoid process, and tenderness along the bicipital groove. Resistance against adduction and flexion of the shoulder caused increased pain over the coracoid process. Although anteroposterior and lateral radiographs of the shoulder were normal, the axillary view showed a fracture through the mid-portion of the base of the coracoid process. Treatment consisted of rest from trap shooting until the patient was asymptomatic, then gradual resumption of activity. Six weeks after the onset of symptoms, the patient had no point tenderness over the coracoid process, and a full, active and painless range of motion of the shoulder. Gradual resumption of shooting caused no shoulder pain, and the patient returned to her usual rate of trap shooting.

The humerus

Stress fracture of the humerus has been described in baseball pitchers,[13–17] a tennis player,[18] a javelin thrower,[19] a bodybuilder,[20] and a weightlifter.[21] Most of the fractures occurred in adolescents and were associated with a recent increase in activity.

Sterling *et al.*[15] report the case of a fourteen-year-old athlete who was competing in swimming and baseball as well as weight training. He felt and heard a 'pop' in his right arm while throwing a baseball. Before the injury occurred, the patient had deep, aching arm pain, and tenderness in the region of the mid shaft of the humerus. Physical examination after the early injury showed swelling, ecchymosis, and extreme pain when arm motion was both active and passive. X-rays revealed a closed comminuted spiral fracture of the humerus that extended proximally. The patient was placed in a cuff and collar for one week, after which a humeral fracture brace was supplied. Three weeks postfracture, the patient had no complaints, and the fracture alignment was anatomic. The pain had ceased about one week earlier. Rehabilitation was instituted by way of an active range of motion, stretching, and progressive-resistance exercises. Six weeks postinjury, radiographs showed abundant callus formation. The brace was removed eleven weeks after the injury occurred, and the patient was allowed to begin swimming. He returned to full activity sixteen weeks postinjury.

Allen[16] describes the case of a thirteen-year-old little-league pitcher who sustained a displaced spiral fracture of the mid humerus while in mid-pitch. The pitcher had had pain in the mid humerus region while at rest, and while pitching during the preceding week. This was presumably a case of a stress fracture that had progressed to an overt fracture during the stress of a ball pitch that involved a forceful side-arm curve.

Branch *et al.*[17] report twelve cases of spontaneous humeral-shaft fractures in a men's over-thirty baseball league. Three-quarters of the pitchers had arm pain at some point before the fracture occurred, and eleven of the twelve heard a crack at the time of the fracture. Nine of the fractures were spiral. Two nerve injuries were associated with the fracture: one injury to the radial and one to the cutaneous nerve. The researchers note four common factors associated with these fractures:
1. age more than thirty years
2. a prolonged period of layoff from pitching
3. lack of a regular exercise program
4. prodromal throwing-arm pain.

Bartsokas *et al.*[20] report the case of a twenty-year-old male bodybuilder who presented with left-shoulder and upper-arm pain that had developed insidiously over a four-week period. Before the onset of pain, the patient had been 'bulking up' for three weeks by lifting heavier than usual weights. Progressive worsening of shoulder and upper-arm pain was reported, particularly when bench presses were undertaken but also by way of incline presses, biceps curls, and overhead presses. Although the symptoms were present only during exercise, they flared up during each weightlifting session, despite one week of rest and treatment with anti-inflammatory medication. Examination revealed mild pain during manual resistance testing of shoulder movements, especially when internal rotation and abduction were undertaken. Mild tenderness to palpation was noted over the insertion of the anterior deltoid muscle. A radiograph revealed a small, lucent line in the cortex of the mid humerus along its anterior aspect. An isotope bone scan showed an area of focal increased activity in the mid-portion of the humerus. The patient was prescribed six weeks' rest followed by gradual resumption of training.

Rettig and Beltz[18] report the case of a fifteen-year-old elite tennis player who had no history of trauma but had a history of onset of pain just above the elbow. The player's symptoms worsened after he began playing more intensively, and he was unable to play for two months because of severe pain. Examination revealed he had full range of motion of the shoulder and elbow and that he had point tenderness over the lateral aspect of the distal third of the humerus. Although early X-rays of the humerus were unremarkable, a bone scan showed abnormal uptake within the ventral aspect of the mid shaft of the humerus. A CT scan showed a vertical fracture through the ventral cortex of the humerus. The patient was instructed to rest for an additional four weeks, then commenced a slow return to tennis. Approximately two weeks after his return, he developed the same pain symptoms. It was therefore believed that his was a case of delayed union, and external electrical stimulation was commenced. His symptoms and signs resolved completely over the following two months, and after a gradual weight-training and flexibility program, he was allowed to return to tennis. He had no more problems. Interestingly, it was noted that the patient was undergoing a growth spurt during the initial occurrence of symptoms and that he had grown some five inches over the five to six months before the onset of symptoms. It was also noted that he was of slight build. It is unclear whether or not this was a true delayed union and therefore whether or not the electrical stimulation affected the healing.

The most probable explanation for occurrence of stress fractures in these younger athletes is that because of the high level of activity among the adolescents, stress was placed on immature bone, and that this was possibly aggravated by a period of rapid growth.

From the few cases of stress fracture of the humerus reported in the literature, the recommended treatment involves a minimum of four weeks' absence from the aggravating activity, then gradual resumption of activity over another four-week period. A strengthening program may be of some benefit.

The olecranon

A small number of stress fractures of the olecranon have been reported, and the diagnosis should be considered in diagnosis of overuse elbow injuries, especially among throwers and gymnasts. The usual presentation is gradual onset of pain in the elbow over a period of a few weeks.

There seem to be three types of stress fracture of the olecranon. The first is a stress fracture of the growth plate, reported in adolescent gymnasts. The fracture appears as a radiolucency extending from the posterior (nonarticular) aspect of the ulna to the articular surface in a transverse manner. Sclerosis of the fracture margins, persistent radiolucency and no relief of pain are signs of delayed or nonunion.[22] The second type is a stress fracture of the tip of the olecranon, seen in throwers, and the third is a stress fracture of the olecranon itself.

Hulkko *et al.*[23] describe cases of four javelin throwers who had a stress fracture of the olecranon. In one of the patients, acute painful dislocation of the fracture occurred during a competitive throw. Two patients had a stress fracture of the tip of the olecranon. One of them was treated conservatively but did not heal for eighteen months. The other patient was treated by excision of the tip and was able to throw after two months. The other two patients had slightly oblique, more distally located stress fractures that were treated with a tension band and two Kirschner wires. The fractures healed in four months. One of the patients had a re-fracture eleven months after the first operation; that

fracture was successfully treated with a compression screw and two bone pegs.

Maffulli *et al.*[24] report two cases of stress fracture through the olecranon growth plate in gymnasts eighteen and nineteen years of age. Conservative management was successful in one case, and the other required internal fixation. The researchers also describe eight younger gymnasts who had traction apophysitis of the olecranon, and postulated that the lesions were probably age dependent. They suggest that when the olecranon apophysis is not fully ossified, traction forces may cause disturbance of blood flow and result in localized areas of avascular necrosis, and disturbed ossification and fragmentation; this is known as traction apophysitis. When the apophysis is more mature but not yet fused, the same forces may produce a stress fracture through the growth plate. Other researchers describe similar stress fractures through the olecranon growth plate.[25–27]

Wilkerson and Johns[28] report a case of nonunion of a stress fracture of the olecranon epiphyseal plate. The fourteen-year-old gymnast first presented with a dull ache and local tenderness. Radiographs revealed a widening of the epiphyseal plate, and diagnosis of stress fracture was made. Three months after discontinuing gymnastics, the patient was found to be asymptomatic and to have a full range of motion. Approximately six months later, the patient returned because of recurrence of pain and limited extension; radiographic evidence showed nonunion. The nonunion site was surgically excised and packed with iliac-crest bone graft. The site was then fixed with a tension-band wire technique, and the patient commenced rehabilitation with emphasis on range-of-motion strengthening. At twelve months postsurgery, the fracture site was completely healed, and range of motion was normal.

Nuber and Diment[29] describe two cases of stress fracture of the olecranon in throwers who were successfully treated by way of conservative methods. Both patients presented with pain around the olecranon that had commenced while they were pitching. They were first diagnosed as having tendonitis, and they continued to pitch until they felt an episode of severe pain during pitching. In both cases, X-rays taken before the episode of acute pain were reported as being normal, whereas X-rays taken after the episode showed evidence of olecranon stress fracture. In one case, the patient was placed in a posterior splint for three weeks. After this, he began elbow range-of-motion and forearm exercises for the following six weeks. Follow-up tomograms undertaken at three months showed evidence of healing, and the patient resumed light throwing. He was able to gradually progress to his previous level of throwing without recurrence of his symptoms. The second patient was prescribed complete rest, until five weeks later, follow-up X-rays showed evidence of fracture healing. The patient continued his activity restriction for two more months, then began exercising and throwing. He returned to his previous level of throwing in six months' time.

Nuber and Diment[29] believe that the transverse stress fracture of the olecranon and the olecranon-tip fractures are not the same entity, even though both fractures were seen in throwers. They state that tip fractures are more likely to be seen in patients who present with a painful elbow after a particularly strong throw. Patients who have a stress fracture, however, are more likely to present with a longer history of pain that recurs when they resume throwing. Radiographically, the tip avulsion fractures involve as much as one-third of the proximal olecranon. The stress fractures occur in the middle third of the olecranon. Tip fractures are likely to go on to nonunion, may form loose bodies, and seem to respond best to surgical incision; olecranon stress fractures, on the other hand, seem to respond to conservative methods.

With reference to stress fractures of the growth plate and of the olecranon itself, if the diagnosis is made relatively early there is a reasonable chance that conservative management could be successful and that the athlete will resume sport in eight to twelve weeks. The treatment of choice for a stress fracture of the tip of the olecranon is surgical excision. Excision would seem to enable the athlete to return to sport at approximately eight weeks.

The ulna

Stress fractures of the ulna have been described in baseball[30,31] and softball[32] pitchers, tennis players,[33–36] volleyball players,[32,37] weight-lifters,[38–41] a ten-pin bowler,[42] and a golfer.[43] Athletes present with pain in the region of the ulna shaft both during and after athletic activity. Physical examination reveals tenderness and pain when movements are undertaken. Radiographs show either a small crack in the cortex of the ulna or a slight haze of new periosteal bone at the stress-fracture site. A bone scan can be used in order to confirm the diagnosis when radiographs fail to show any abnormality. In all the reported cases, the patient returned to activity in four to six weeks after a period of rest from the aggravating activity, and after gradual resumption of activity.

Mutoh *et al.*[32] describe stress fractures of the ulna in a softball pitcher who was throwing underarm, and in a volleyball player who experienced pain during underhand maneuvers. Both actions involved repetitive movements of the unilateral upper limb when a light load was applied after contraction of the flexor muscles. In the volleyball player, who had more-pronounced wrist flexion, the stress was more proximal; in the softball player, it was more distal.

Bollen *et al.*[33] describe two stress fractures of the ulna in tennis players. In the first case, a seventeen-year-old, right-handed, female, professional-tennis player complained of gradually increasing pain in the left forearm when she was using the double-handed backhand stroke. The only physical findings were tenderness over the middle third of the ulna, and pain when pronation was resisted. Although radiographs were unremarkable, an isotope bone scan showed markedly increased uptake over the tenderness site (Fig. 6.1).

In the second case, a 21-year-old, right-handed, male, professional-tennis player also complained of pain in the left forearm. He had been undertaking intensive backhand training over the preceding few weeks, and had developed increasing pain over the anteromedial aspect of the forearm during ball contact when he was using the double-handed backhand stroke. He also had tenderness to palpation of the anteromedial aspect of the ulna at the junction of the proximal and middle thirds. Although radiographs were normal, the presence of a stress fracture was confirmed by way of a bone scan. Both patients were treated by way of standard procedures for stress fractures: resting of the affected limb, and gradual resumption of activities after resolution of the tenderness.

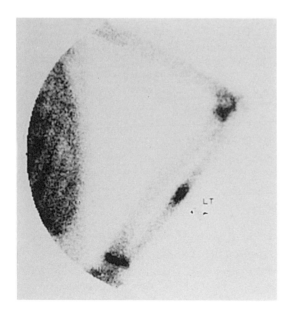

Fig. 6.1
An isotope bone scan of a stress fracture of the ulnar diaphysis.

The researchers believe that the injury mechanism was similar to that reported in softball players by Tanabe *et al.*:[37] repetitive excessive pronation. In tennis players' double-handed backhand stroke, pronation occurs during the phase of ball strike and follow-through, and presumably causes torsional stresses similar to the ones found in the softball players. Young *et al.*[34] report the similar case of a fifteen-year-old female tennis player.

Bell and Hawkins[36] describe the case of a nineteen-year-old right-handed tennis player who presented with left-wrist pain that had commenced while he was hitting a two-handed backhand. He described the pain as being just proximal to the ulnar styloid, and it involved both the dorsal and the volar aspects of the forearm. He was tender to palpation along the ulnar aspect of the distal forearm. Direct palpation of the distal third of the ulna, three to four centimeters proximal to the ulnar styloid, reproduced pain similar to that encountered during backhands. Marked dorsiflexion of the wrist, and pronation–supination, also elicited pain. Plain X-rays of the forearm revealed a discrete area of periosteal elevation along the dorsal aspect of the distal ulna. Diagnosis of stress fracture was made, and treatment consisted of a modification of the patient's swing pattern and an attempt to use a one-handed backhand. A dorsally applied extension-block splint was applied on a temporary basis. After four weeks, the patient returned to his full level of activity and resumed his two-handed backhand, pain free at that point. Repeat X-rays at the time showed additional callus.

Escher[42] describes the case of a sixteen-year-old right-handed bowler who reported three weeks of increasing pain in the proximal right ulna. The young man bowled three to eight games per day using a 16 pound, fingertip ball. An isotope bone scan showed increased uptake in the ulna in his area of pain. Management consisted of five weeks' bowling cessation and gradual return to activity. The researcher postulates that the fracture was caused by stress on the ulna at the origin of the flexor profundus muscle from repeatedly grasping the ball by way of fingertip grip.

Koskinen *et al.*[43] report the case of a 44-year-old golfer who presented with a four-week history of a painful left wrist. In the report, it is not mentioned whether the golfer was right or left handed. Radiographs showed a periosteal reaction on the radial side of the distal ulnar diaphysis. An MRI disclosed cortical thickening and an area of low signal density on T1-weighted images, as well as edema on T2-weighted images, consistent with a healing stress fracture. One week later, radiographs showed a lucent fracture line with periosteal callus. The patient's golf instructor recognized that the affected left hand used excessive external rotation.

The radius

Stress fracture of the radius was first described in the military setting. Farquharson-Roberts and Fulford[44] described a case in which a 23-year-old naval recruit developed bilateral radial stress fractures after training or 'field gun running', an activity in which the person catches a heavy gun barrel across his or her forearms and handles a heavy gun over simulated obstacles. Radiographs showed stress fractures of the radius bilaterally in the proximal third along the anterior cortex. Treatment consisted of six weeks' rest, and progressive return to training. No complications were reported, and radiographically the fractures seemed to be well healed six weeks later.

Stress fractures of the radius have also been described in gymnasts,[45–47] a tennis player,[48] a pool player,[49] and a cyclist.[50] Stress injuries of the distal radial growth plate are seen frequently in young gymnasts.[45,47]

Ahluwalia *et al.*[46] describe the case of a 24-year-old female gymnast who had a three-month history of bilateral forearm pain. The pain began when the gymnast increased her training from nine to eighteen hours per week. Radiographs showed no abnormality, but an isotope bone scan revealed focally increased activity in the radial shafts, in both arms.

Eisenberg *et al.*[50] report the case of a twelve-year-old boy who presented with a three-week history of pain in the left wrist and forearm. He stated that he had been riding a bicycle very hard for several months, and doing 'wheelies' by jerking the bike's front wheel off the ground and riding on the back wheel only. The front wheel then came back down to the ground with a hard thud, thereby jarring his forearm. The left forearm was tender at the junction of the mid and distal thirds of the radius, and X-rays revealed a fracture line at the distal radial diaphysis, and periosteal new-bone formation.

Loosli and Leslie[48] describe the case of a 25-year-old, high-level, right-handed, female tennis player who developed increasing pain in her right wrist. Physical examination revealed diffuse tenderness of the distal radius and over the second and third metacarpals dorsally. Hyperextension of the wrist caused pain at the back of the hand, and extension of the thumb to resistance caused pain to the back of the hand and wrist, as well as pain in the proximal second and third metacarpals. Although X-rays were normal, a bone scan showed markedly increased uptake in the distal radius. At the time of diagnosis, the player had had persistent pain for five months despite reduced activity undertaken using a splint. She was therefore placed in a short arm cast for three weeks, then a posterior splint for three more weeks. When the posterior splint was applied, she began an isometric strengthening program for her wrist flexors and extensors. After her immobilization, she began a strengthening program of resistive exercise using latex tubing. She began hitting the tennis ball painlessly approximately eight weeks after immobilization was commenced. She gradually progressed to painless tennis on alternate days, and in two and a half months she was able to hit a tennis ball comfortably. She returned to painless, full, competitive-level tennis at three months.

Orloff and Resnick[49] report the case of a 22-year-old pool player who complained of a painful mass on the dorsum of the distal part of the right forearm. The pain was accentuated when the forearm was rotated in a movement designed to 'put English' on the billiards ball. The patient spent at least four consecutive hours playing pool three nights per week. Radiographs showed fluffy periosteal reaction extending 2 centimeters along the dorso-ulnar margin of the distal third of the radius. Sixteen weeks later, the pain had subsided, and radiographs revealed a healing stress fracture.

The scaphoid

A stress fracture of the scaphoid combined with distal radial epiphysiolysis has been reported.[51] In the report, a sixteen-year-old badminton player who practiced three hours per day, six days per week, presented with a seven-week history of wrist pain. His pain was brought on by forced passive dorsiflexion and volarflexion of the wrist. A semipronated oblique radiograph showed a nondisplaced fracture through the waist of the scaphoid, and widening of the distal radial epiphysis. The wrist was immobilized in a short thumb-spica cast for eight weeks, and there was good radiographic healing.

Of the five other cases of stress fracture of the scaphoid reported in the literature, four were of gymnasts and one was of a shotputter.[52,53] All the activities involve repeated wrist movements, mainly dorsiflexion. The fractures were all nondisplaced transverse fractures of the scaphoid waist, including sclerotic borders, and all were well managed by way of immobilization in a thumb-spica cast.

The metacarpal

A total of eight cases of metacarpal stress fractures are reported in the literature; five were in sportspeople, and three were related to occupation. The stress fractures related to occupation involved the second metacarpal, and resulted from extrinsic pressure from a solid object such as an ice-cream scoop[54] or a pen,[55] whereby a force was exerted on the second metacarpal.

Details are available about three of the five reported stress fractures of the metacarpal in athletes; the other two fractures were reported as part of a large series.[56] Two of the athlete cases involved stress fracture of the second metacarpal bone in tennis players;[57,58] the third case involved a stress fracture of the fifth metacarpal in a softball pitcher.[59]

Similarities exist between the metacarpal and metatarsal bones. The second metacarpal is the longest and has the largest base of all the metacarpals; it articulates at the base with the trapezoid, trapezium, capitate, and third metacarpal. Movement at the second carpo-metacarpal joint is limited in directions other than flexion–extension. The fifth metacarpal articulates with other bones only on the lateral aspect of the base with the fourth metacarpal and hamate, whereas its medial surface is nonarticular and presents a tubercle for insertion of extensor carpi ulnaris. The conformation of its base allows for a range of motion greater than that of the second, third, and fourth metacarpals in directions other than flexion–extension. In the metatarsal bones, it is probable that the relative frequency of stress fractures of the second metatarsal reflects the bone's immobility at the base, whereas the fifth metatarsal articulates at only part of its base and has insertion from the powerful peroneus brevis tendon.

As is the case with so many stress fractures, the precipitating factors in development of the three described metacarpal stress fractures are a combination of increased load and technique changes. In the two cases of stress fracture of the second metacarpal in tennis players,[57,58] the players described an increase in training volume and intensity as well as an alteration in technique. Intrinsic pressure from a solid object, the racquet, on the second metacarpal bone provides a fulcrum for an external compressive load.[60]

The softball player who presented with a stress fracture of the fifth metacarpal (Fig. 6.2) had recently increased her training intensity in preparation for a major competition, and had altered the grip for her curve ball. This involved an increased amount of abduction of the fifth finger, and ball delivery using the fingers perpendicular to the pitch direction, thereby increasing abduction forces.[59]

In all the described cases of stress fracture of the metacarpals, relative rest and avoidance of aggravating activity resulted in clinical healing within four weeks. Attention must be paid to the technique errors and training overload that first precipitate the problem.

SUMMARY

- Stress fractures of the upper limb are infrequent but not rare.
- The literature case reports summarized in this chapter probably represent only a small proportion of all upper-limb stress fractures.
- Upper-limb stress fractures are examples of bone-stress injuries as a result of repetitive muscle pull.
- Diagnosis of stress fracture should always be considered in overuse syndromes of the upper limb.
- Careful anatomic examination is required.
- If localized bony tenderness is present, the clinician should suspect stress fracture.
- A plain radiograph should be performed. However, if it is negative, when clinical symptoms and signs indicate possible stress fracture the clinician should immediately proceed to isotope bone scan.
- Upper-limb stress fractures generally heal when the athlete has rest from the aggravating activity.
- Technique problems have to be addressed before the athlete returns to his or her sport.

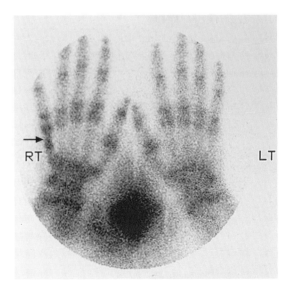

Fig. 6.2
An isotope bone scan of a stress fracture of the fifth metacarpal.

References

1   Cummings CW, First R. Stress fracture of the clavicle after a radical neck dissection. *Plastic and Reconstructive Surgery* 1975; 55: 366–367.

2   Ord RA, Langdon JD. Stress fracture of the clavicle: a rare late complication of radical neck dissection. *Journal of Maxillofacial Surgery* 1986; 24: 281–284.

3   Adolfsson L, Lysholm J. Case report: clavicular stress fracture in a javelin thrower. *Clinics in Sports Medicine* 1990; 2: 41–45.

4   Waninger KN. Stress fracture of the clavicle in a collegiate diver. *Clinical Journal of Sport Medicine* 1997; 7: 66–68.

5   Nagy E, Szabo L, Nagy Z. Fatigue fracture of the scapula. *Monattschr Unfallheilkd* 1967; 70: 63.

6   Mandak P, Wondrak E. Unusual fatigue fracture of the scapula with rupture of the biceps muscle. *Acta Chirurgie Traumatologie Czech* 1972; 39: 295.

7   Ho SC, Hsu SYC, Leung PC *et al.* A longitudinal study of the determinants of bone mass in Chinese women aged 21–40. *Annals of Epidemiology* 1993; 3: 256–263.

8   Brower AC, Neff AR, Tillema DA. An unusual scapula stress fracture. *American Journal of Radiology* 1977; 129: 519–520.

9   Nagle CE, Freitas JE. Radionuclide imaging of musculoskeletal injuries in athletes with negative radiographs. *Physician and Sportsmedicine* 1987; 15: 147–155.

10 Veluvolu P, Kolen HS, Guten GN *et al.* Unusual stress fracture of the scapula in a jogger. *Clinical Nuclear Medicine* 1988; 13 (7): 531–532.

11 Ward WG, Bergfeld JA, Carson WG. Stress fracture of the base of the acromial process. *American Journal of Sports Medicine* 1994; 22 (1): 146–147.

12 Boyer DWJ. Trapshooter's shoulder: stress fractures of the coracoid process – case report. *Journal of Bone and Joint Surgery* 1975; 57A: 862.

13 Herzmark MH, Clune FR. Ball-throwing fracture of the humerus. *Medical Annals of District of Columbia* 1952; 21: 196–199.

14 Devas M. *Stress fractures*. London: Churchill Livingstone, 1975.

15 Sterling JC, Calvo RD, Holden SC. An unusual stress fracture in a multiple sport athlete. *Medicine and Science in Sports and Exercise* 1991; 23: 298–303.

16 Allen ME. Stress fracture of the humerus: a case study. *American Journal of Sports Medicine* 1984; 12: 244–245.

17 Branch T, Partin C, Chamberland P, Emeterio E, Sabetelle M. Spontaneous fractures of the humerus during pitching: a series of 12 cases. *American Journal of Sports Medicine* 1992; 20: 468–470.

18 Rettig AC, Beltz HF. Stress fracture in the humerus in an adolescent tennis tournament player. *American Journal of Sports Medicine* 1985; 13 (1): 55–58.

19 Hartley JB. 'Stress' or 'fatigue' fractures of bone. *British Journal of Radiology* 1943; 16: 255–262.

20 Bartsokas TW, Palin WD, Collier BD. An unusual stress fracture site: mid humerus. *Physician and Sportsmedicine* 1992; 20 (2): 119–122.

21 Horwitz BR, DiStefano V. Stress fracture of the humerus in a weight lifter. *Orthopedics* 1995; 18 (2): 185–187.

22 Hershman EB, Mailly T. Stress fractures. *Clinics in Sports Medicine* 1990; 9: 183–241.

23 Hulkko A, Orava S, Nikula P. Stress fractures of the olecranon in javelin throwers. *International Journal of Sports Medicine* 1986; 7: 210–213.

24 Maffulli N, Chan D, Aldridge MJ. Overuse injuries of the olecranon in young gymnasts. *Journal of Bone and Joint Surgery* 1992; 74 (2): 305–308.

25 Torg JS, Moyer RA. Non-union of a stress fracture through the olecranon epiphyseal plate observed in an adolescent baseball pitcher: a case report. *Journal of Bone and Joint Surgery* 1977; 59A: 264–265.

26 Pavlov H, Torg JS, Jacobs B, Vigorita V. Nonunion of olecranon epiphysis: two cases in adolescent baseball pitchers. *American Journal of Roentgenology* 1981; 136: 819–820.

27 Retrum RK, Wepfer JF, Olen DW, Laney WH. Case report 355: delayed closure of the right olecranon epiphysis in a right handed tournament class tennis player (post-traumatic). *Skeletal Radiology* 1986; 15: 185–187.

28 Wilkerson RD, Johns JC. Nonunion of an olecranon stress fracture in an adolescent gymnast: a case report. *American Journal of Sports Medicine* 1990; 18: 432–434.

29 Nuber GW, Diment MT. Olecranon stress fractures in throwers: a report of two cases and a review of the literature. *Clinical Orthopaedics and Related Research* 1992; 278: 58–61.

30 Feinberg JH, Davis BA. Occult ulnar fracture in a high school pitcher. *American Medical Society for Sports Medicine – 3rd Annual Meeting*. Rancho Mirage, California, 1994: 1.

31 Pascale MS, Grana WA. Answer please: stress fracture of the ulna. *Orthopedics* 1988; 11 (5): 829–832.

32 Mutoh Y, Mori T, Suzuki Y, Sugiura Y. Stress fractures of the ulna in athletes. *American Journal of Sports Medicine* 1982; 10: 365–367.

33 Bollen SR, Robinson DG, Crichton KJ, Cross MJ. Stress fractures of the ulna in tennis players using a double-handed backhand stroke. *American Journal of Sports Medicine* 1993; 21: 751–752.

34 Young CC, Raasch WG, Geiser C. Ulnar stress fracture of the nondominant arm in a tennis player using a two-handed backhand. *Clinical Journal of Sport Medicine* 1995; 5: 262–264.

35 Rettig AC. Stress fracture of the ulna in an adolescent tournament tennis player. *American Journal of Sports Medicine* 1983; 11: 103–109.

36 Bell RH, Hawkins RJ. Stress fracture of the distal ulna: a case report. *Clinical Orthopaedics and Related Research* 1986; 209: 169–171.

37 Tanabe S, Nakahira J, Bando E *et al.* Fatigue fracture of the ulna occurring in pitchers of fast-pitch softball. *American Journal of Sports Medicine* 1991; 19: 317–321.

38 Hamilton KH. Stress fracture of the diaphysis of the ulna in a body builder. *American Journal of Sports Medicine* 1984; 12: 405–406.

39 Patel MR, Irizarry J, Stricevic M. Stress fracture of the ulna diaphysis: review of the literature and report of a case. *Journal of Hand Surgery (Am)* 1986; 11 (3): 443–445.

40 Heinricks EH, Senske BJ. Stress fracture of the ulna diaphysis in athletes: a case report and review of the literature. *South Dakota Journal of Medicine* 1988; 41 (2): 5–8.

41 Chen WC, Hsu WY, Wu JJ. Stress fracture of the diaphysis of the ulna. *International Orthopaedics* 1991; 15 (3): 197–198.

42 Escher SA. Ulnar diaphyseal stress fracture in a bowler. *American Journal of Sports Medicine* 1997; 25 (3): 412–413.

43 Koskinen SK, Mattila KT, Alanen AM, Aro HT. Stress fracture of the ulnar diaphysis in a recreational golfer. *Clinical Journal of Sport Medicine* 1997; 7: 63–65.

44 Farquharson-Roberts MA, Fulford PC. Stress fracture of the radius. *Journal of Bone and Joint Surgery* 1980; 62-B: 194–195.

45 Carter SR, Aldridge MJ. Stress injury of the distal radial growth plate. *Journal of Bone and Joint Surgery* 1988; 70 (5): 834–836.

46 Ahluwalia R, Datz FL, Morton KA, Anderson CM, Whiting JHJ. Bilateral fatigue fractures of the radial shaft in a gymnast. *Clinics in Nuclear Medicine* 1994; 19 (8): 665–667.

47 Read MTF. Stress fracture of the distal radius in adolescent gymnasts. *British Journal of Sports Medicine* 1981; 15 (4): 272–276.

48 Loosli AR, Leslie M. Stress fractures of the distal radius. *American Journal of Sports Medicine* 1991; 19 (5): 523–524.

49 Orloff AS, Resnick D. Fatigue fracture of the distal part of the radius in a pool player. *British Journal of Accident Surgery* 1986; 17 (6): 418–419.

50 Eisenberg D, Kirchner SG, Green NE. Stress fracture of the distal radius caused by 'wheelies'. *Southern Medical Journal* 1986; 79 (7): 918–919.

51 Inagaki H, Inoue G. Stress fracture of the scaphoid combined with distal radial epiphysiolysis. *British Journal of Sports Medicine* 1997; 31: 256–257.

52 Mazione M, Pizzutillo PD. Stress fracture of the scaphoid waist: a case report. *American Journal of Sports Medicine* 1981; 9: 268–269.

53 Hanks GA, Kalenak A, Bowman LS, Sebastianelli WJ. Stress fractures of the carpal scaphoid. *Journal of Bone and Joint Surgery (Am)* 1989; 71: 938–941.

54 Howard RS II, Conrad GR. Ice cream scooper's hand: report of an occupationally related stress fracture of the hand. *Clinical Nuclear Medicine* 1992; 17 (9): 721–723.

55 Gokturk E, Vardareli E, Gunal I, Seber S. Metacarpal stress fracture in an accountant. *Acta Orthopedica Scandinavica* 1995; 66 (3): 295.

56 Orava S, Hulkko A. Delayed unions and nonunions of stress fractures in athletes. *American Journal of Sports Medicine* 1988; 16: 378–382.

57 Murakami Y. Stress fracture of the metacarpal in an adolescent tennis player. *American Journal of Sports Medicine* 1988; 16: 419–420.

58 Waninger KN, Lombardo JA. Stress fracture of index metacarpal in an adolescent tennis player. *Clinical Journal of Sport Medicine* 1995; 5 (1): 63–66.

59 Jowett A, Brukner P. Fifth metacarpal stress fracture in a female softball pitcher. *Clinical Journal of Sport Medicine* 1997; 7: 220–221.

60 Plagehoef S. Tennis racket testing related to tennis elbow. In: Groppel J, ed. *A National Symposium on the Racket Sports.* Urbana-Champaign: University of Illinois Press, 1979: 291–310.

Chapter 7

Stress fractures of the trunk

In the trunk, the most commonly seen stress fractures are those of the lower ribs and the pars interarticularis. Less commonly reported stress fractures occur in the sternum, first rib, and sacrum.

The sternum

In the literature, three cases of stress fracture of the sternum have been reported: one in a wrestler,[1] one in a golfer,[2] and one in a body-builder.[3] All three fractures were associated with a recent increase in activity and gradual onset of pain over the sternum. Isotope bone scan showed a focal region of increased uptake at the pain site. The symptoms resolved over a three- to four-week period, during which activity was reduced.

The first rib

Stress fracture of the first rib is more common than is realized and should be considered in differential diagnosis of shoulder, mid scapular and clavicular pain.

Two types of 'stress fracture' of the first rib are seen in athletes. The first type is an acute fracture for which onset of pain is sudden, and the second is a 'true' stress fracture for which onset of pain is gradual. Some researchers[4,5] describe the acute fracture as a stress fracture, presumably because they assume that the bone has previously been weakened by repeated stress and that a particularly severe stress causes an acute fracture. However, in most of the cases no symptoms were present before the acute fracture occurred, so we are reluctant to consider these to be true stress fractures.

The one reported exception is the case described by Lankenner and Micheli,[6] in which a fifteen-year-old boy who had been active in little-league baseball for seven years had dull, aching pain in the posterior aspect of his right shoulder twenty-four hours before an acute fracture occurred when he tried to swing a bat. Radiographs of the right shoulder showed an apparent fracture of the right first rib, and the diagnosis was confirmed using isotope bone scan. The boy had undergone a rapid increase in quantity and intensity of training over a four-week period before the onset of symptoms; therefore, the injury could probably be viewed as being an acute fracture through a stress-fracture site. The boy returned to baseball after four weeks.

Rademaker *et al.*[7] report two cases of first-rib stress fracture. The first case is that of a 21-year-old mother who presented with continuous shoulder and clavicular pain that was exacerbated when she inspired. Although she had not received direct trauma to her shoulder, her history indicated a link between the onset of pain and lifting her two-year-old daughter. Diagnosis was confirmed by way of a chest radiograph. The second case is that of a fourteen-year-old girl who had a three-week history of left-shoulder and scapular pain that was exacerbated when she inspired deeply. The onset of pain coincided with a period of strenuous work to which the girl was unaccustomed. Examination revealed no abnormalities, and the diagnosis was confirmed by way of chest radiography.

Sacchetti *et al.*[8] describe two cases of first-rib 'stress fracture' in young basketball players. The first case is that of a fracture of sudden onset, and the second case was that of a fifteen-year-old boy who described right-shoulder pain that he had first noticed when he was rapidly abducting his arms during a basketball game. Physical examination revealed marked point tenderness to palpation immediately inferior to the mid-point of the clavicle, and radiographic examination revealed a nondisplaced fracture of the first rib anteriorly.

Mintz *et al.*[9] describe the case of a nineteen-year-old right-handed man who had had gradual onset of pain after completing a workout on an exercise machine. The man had concluded a set of upper-body 'flies' (arm abduction against resistance in the horizontal plane) using 100 pounds of resistance. The man had then had a partner forcibly abduct the man's arms against maximal resistance, and had immediately afterward noticed 'muscle stiffness' in the left-scapular region. Over the rest of the day, the pain in the left-posterior shoulder increased and radiated along the ulnar aspect of the left arm to the little finger. Physical examination revealed point tenderness medial to the superior angle of the left scapula. A chest radiograph revealed a complete transverse minimally displaced fracture of the left first rib at the junction of the posterior and middle thirds. The patient was immobilized in a sling for ten days, and two months later he had no discomfort. Repeat radiographs showed callus formation.

Crichton *et al.*[10] describe five cases of stress fracture of the first rib in ballet dancers, and one of the fractures was bilateral. The researchers concluded that ballet dancers and people who lift and throw heavy weights above their shoulders have an increased risk of this type of fracture.

The typical presentation for stress fracture of the first rib is gradual onset of unilateral shoulder and medial scapular pain that is aggravated by deep inspiration and coughing. There is usually either a history of increased activity or some change in type of activity. When the person is examined, there is invariably local tenderness over the first rib. In all the reported cases, the fracture was visible on an anteroposterior chest radiograph (Fig. 7.1). Isotope bone scan also shows a focal area of increased activity in the first rib (Fig. 7.2).

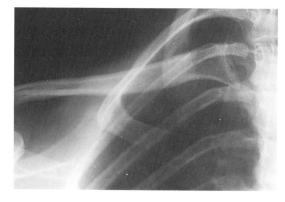

Fig. 7.1
A radiograph of a stress fracture of the first rib.

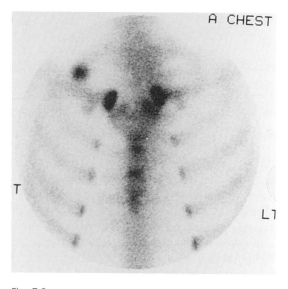

Fig. 7.2
An isotope bone scan of a stress fracture of the first rib.

For the true stress fractures described, all the patients were treated by having four weeks' rest from the aggravating activity, and all fully recovered. No acute neurovascular complications have been reported, and none of the late complications that are seen in traumatic fractures of the first rib have been identified, such as Horner's syndrome and late thoracic outlet syndrome. For traumatic fractures of the first rib, a relatively high incidence of delayed union or nonunion has been described, a nonpainful pseudoarthrosis has occasionally developed. Ochi *et al.*[11] describe a case of brachial-plexus palsy caused by a stress fracture of the first rib, in a thirteen-year-old volleyball player. The palsy was apparently caused by pressure exerted through excessive callus formation following nonunion. Although conservative treatment was unsuccessful, surgical decompression led to complete resolution of the symptoms.

Most fractures of the first rib are located in an area of relative anatomic weakness: a shallow groove at which the subclavian artery crosses the rib.[12,13] The rib is rigidly attached posteriorly and anteriorly, and there are multiple muscle attachments to the region. The scalenus anterior inserts on the scalene tubercle of the first rib between the subclavian artery and vein, and provides a cephalad pull. The serratus anterior attaches to the same region, but on the inferior surface, and Sacchetti *et al.*[8] suggest that the fracture was the result of contraction of muscles the forces of which act in opposing directions. They postulated that combined with the downward pull of the serratus anterior, the upward pull of the scalenus anterior caused an adequate force to produce a fracture of the point of maximal stress, which is commonly the area just posterior to the scalene tubercle.

In the abovementioned case described by Mintz *et al.*,[9] in which a stress fracture of the rib was sustained while an exercise machine was being used, the maneuvers used on the exercise machine were re-created by way of magnetic resonance images that were acquired before and after exercise. In this injury, the T2 changes in the serratus anterior muscle supported involvement of serratus anterior as the main muscle that acted on the first rib.

In two of the cases of first-rib stress fracture described among ballet dancers by Crichton *et al.*,[10] the dancers participated in sequences that involved lifting the dancers' partner. They had been involved in technique changes that specifically involved shoulder depression. The researchers commented on serratus anterior's role in protracting the scapula in punching or pushing movements. The muscle also powerfully helps the trapezius in rotating the scapula laterally and upward in raising the arm above the level of the shoulder. In their routine, the dancers are likely to have thrown their partner, and throwing is both a pushing movement and a movement for which the arms have to be lifted above the shoulder.

It would seem that excessive action of the serratus anterior muscle either alone or as opposed by the scalenes leads to a stress fracture of the first rib.

The lower ribs

Stress fractures of the ribs have been described in golfers,[14–23] rowers,[16,24–26] paddlers,[27] tennis players,[16] gymnasts,[16] squash players,[28] and a swimmer.[29]

Lord and Carson[17] describe the case of a 36-year-old right-handed man who had recently taken up golf. On the practise range, the man hit two buckets of golfballs per day six or seven days per week, for about eight weeks. Pain gradually developed in the left posterior thoracic region, beneath his scapula. He was at first diagnosed as having thoracic back strain, and seven months later his symptoms had almost resolved when he developed an upper-respiratory illness and the coughing reactivated his back pain.

When he was examined, although he had no palpable tenderness he had mild crepitation between his left scapula and thoracic ribs. A bone scan revealed increased uptake on the posterolateral aspects of the left sixth, seventh, and eighth ribs that was consistent with stress fracture. Plain radiographs suggested these were healing fractures. After six weeks of relative rest, the man's pain improved. He began a strengthening program in which the focus was on increasing the endurance of the serratus anterior, rhomboid, levator scapulae and trapezius muscles. Four weeks later, his symptoms subsided and he gradually returned to playing golf. He remained asymptomatic and continued to play golf once a week. The researchers postulated that the mechanism of injury may be the result of fatigue of the serratus anterior, and that this may then lead to glenohumeral–scapulothoracic asynchrony.

Orava *et al.*[19] describe five cases of stress fracture of the rib in middle-aged novice golfers. All the subjects were right-handed players and in four of the five cases the stress fracture was on the right-hand side. The fractures were usually located anterolaterally, and the ribs involved were the third, sixth and seventh. All the patients presented with chest pain on the side of the fracture and in most cases were originally thought to have either an intercostal muscle strain or Tietze's syndrome. In all the cases, a chest radiograph showed a clear stress fracture in the mid axillary line. The patients were advised to rest from golf for three to six weeks, and all of them were able to resume their activity. The researchers postulated that in golf, the mechanism of rib stress fractures is probably force exerted by contraction of the serratus and abdominal muscles, contraction of the latissimus dorsi, and bending of the upper body during the swing phase, including possible impingement on the thoracic cage and ribs of the right side.

Lord *et al.*[22] conducted a retrospective review that involved three institutions, and documented nineteen cases of rib stress fractures in golfers.

There were thirteen men and six women, and the average age was thirty-nine years. Eighteen of the golfers were beginners, and before his injury occurred, the one experienced golfer had dramatically increased his practise time on the driving range. The beginners had been playing golf for an average of eight weeks before they presented for medical evaluation. All the fractures occurred along the posterolateral aspect of the ribs, ten of the patients sustained a single-rib fracture, and nine of the patients sustained multiple rib fractures. Fifteen sustained injury on the leading side of the trunk, three sustained injury on the trailing side, and one sustained bilateral rib fractures. The fourth to the sixth were the most commonly involved ribs. Plain radiographs, including oblique views for rib detail, showed the fractures in sixteen of the patients, and in the other three cases isotope bone scan was necessary for diagnosis.

Read[20] reports the case of a 45-year-old, nine-handicap, right-handed golfer who had played golf for 13 years, and had presented with a one-month history of acute onset of right anterior chest pain experienced while playing golf. Five months earlier, he had had one episode of similar pain when hitting a fairway wood, and that pain had resolved after had a six-week rest from golf. He had had no more trouble until the new episode. Although he had been treated elsewhere for thoracic vertebral dysfunction, clinically he had a full and painless range of neck and thoracic movements, and rib spring was positive over the 5/6 anterior axillary line. Fracture of the right fifth rib was confirmed by way of isotope bone scan. Radiography showed a healing fracture and no other pathology. The researcher stated that although the golfer was a 'hooker' of the ball, he would block the shot when he failed to rotate through the ball, by sliding his right side under and hitting with his body before his hands. He was able to reproduce some discomfort with this swing, even when his normal swing, with full rotation through the shot, was pain free. The researcher believed it was possible that rowers have a similar problem whereby rather than pull with the inside hand (the hand further away from the blade) and produce a rotation of the dorsal spine, they pulled too soon with the feathering outside hand, and thereby blocked this rotation.

Orava *et al.*[28] describe the case of a seventeen-year-old boy who had played squash for five years. Over the preceding year, he had played about twenty hours per week. He described a history of right-thoracic pain that was provoked by either coughing or playing over the preceding ten days. Before the symptoms had occurred, he had changed his training by increasing the number of hits and increasing the rotational movements of his trunk during the hits. When he was examined, he was tender on the right thorax at the anterior axillary line. The first radiograph showed a fissure across the seventh rib laterally. Two weeks later, fusiform callus formation was seen at the fracture site. After about five weeks' rest and modified training, the patient resumed playing squash, and was asymptomatic.

Holden and Jackson[16] describe seven stress fractures, four of which were in rowers, and one each of which was in a tennis player, a golf player and a gymnast. All four rowers were female, were engaged at an elite level of rowing, and were training specifically for single sculling. Each athlete had been examined elsewhere, and had had a diagnosis of muscular strain. The time from onset of symptoms to diagnosis ranged from two weeks to six months. In all the cases, bone scans and/or radiographs were used for making the diagnosis.

Brukner and Khan[25] describe a case of stress fracture in an elite sculler. The interesting aspect of the case is that the fracture was located posteriorly (Fig. 7.3), close to the costovertebral junction, rather than laterally, as was the case with all other described rib stress fractures.

Taimela *et al.*[29] report the case of a 21-year-old female swimmer who had participated in competitive swimming for five years, and who

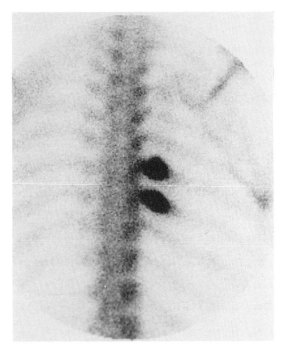

Fig. 7.3
An isotope bone scan that shows an unusual posterior stress fracture of the seventh and eighth ribs.

had trained for 20 to 25 hours per week over the preceding year. The young woman's training consisted of freestyle swimming, weight training, and running. She described an initial period of chest pain that had lasted for three months and had forced her to cease training for several weeks. It had been believed that the pain was of muscular origin, and no radiograph had been taken. The pain had gradually settled, and the young woman had trained for twelve months without experiencing symptoms. She had then developed poorly localized minimal pain on the right side of the thorax, below the scapula. After one month, she had heard an abnormal cracking sound during a stretching exercise, and the thoracic pain had become sharp and constant. Clinical examination revealed that the patient had pain during palpation of the right side of the thorax, below the scapula in the region of the ninth rib. Protuberances were felt in the fifth and ninth ribs. The initial radiograph showed old callus posteriorly across the somewhat distorted fifth rib posteriorly. Three weeks later, a fracture line and callus formation were seen at the ninth rib. After having approximately four weeks' rest and undertaking modified training, the patient resumed swimming, and at six weeks was asymptomatic.

Various theories have been proposed for the mechanism of injury for rib stress fractures.[16] Seilin[30] and Tunis[31] consider the diaphragm to be the most likely cause of stress fractures, combined with muscular groups such as the latissimus dorsi or external oblique muscles. Oechsli[32] believes that the diaphragm cannot be the key muscle, because it has no specific anatomic attachment that correlates with the location of most rib fractures. He suggests that opposing forces of the serratus anterior and external oblique muscles are more likely to create fractures by way of their attachment near the site of the rib fractures found in his series.

Derbes and Harran[14] analyzed the structural characteristics of a rib, and the muscular forces involved, by using free-body diagrams. They predicted the rib areas that would undergo the greatest bending, shear, tensile, and compressive stresses, and found that most rib fractures do, in fact, occur at the location of the highest predicted bending stress. This point corresponds with the rib's posterolateral segments, and was the location of the fractures described in most cases in the literature. Because of its significant anatomic muscular attachment to the ribs, the serratus anterior is one of the major contributors to bending stresses across the rib. Satou and Konisi[33] undertook biomechanical studies of the sixth rib, and found that compression and tension stresses are greatest on the posterolateral segments.

It would therefore seem that any upper-extremity movement that involves the serratus anterior and force couples such as the major and minor rhomboids could exert significant stress across the ribs posterolaterally. Holden and Jackson[16] describe how this movement occurs during the rowing maneuver. During the first part of the rowing stroke, the drive phase, angular velocity is generated through use of the legs and a stiffened torso. In this phase, the scapula muscles contract isometrically, and thereby transmit the torso's power to the arms. However, the end of the drive involves drawing of the hands toward the body, in association with shoulder extension and scapular retraction. The rhomboids, trapezius and serratus anterior act isotonically, and thereby pull the scapula in a controlled way along the rib cage posteriorly toward the mid-line. This maneuver is accentuated in sculling as opposed to sweep rowing, because there is less body torsion, and a greater range of motion is available at the shoulders, because each arm separately controls the oar. During the recovery, the scapula is pulled anteriorly by the main protractor, the serratus anterior, while the rest of the shoulder is flexed and the elbow is extended. Similar stresses seemed to be applied during the two weight-training exercises of bench press and bench pull, which are commonly undertaken by rowers.

Holden and Jackson[16] note that all four of their scullers who had developed a rib stress fracture were female. They postulate that most women involved in competition in which the upper extremity is involved basically lack a strength-training background, and are therefore at increased risk of developing a rib fracture when using high-pressure resistance-training techniques in mainly upper-extremity sports.

Christiansen and Kanstrup[26] report that six cases of rib stress fracture occurred among national female and male elite rowers over a period of fourteen months.

As is the case with all stress fractures, in all the cases described a rapid increase in activity seems to be a precipitating factor. The symptoms of rib stress fracture are mainly pain associated with activity, especially any activity that involves twisting. The problem is frequently misdiagnosed as being an intercostal muscle strain.

Clinicians should have a high suspicion of rib stress fracture for any athlete who presents with these symptoms. An oblique radiograph should be obtained, and in many cases it will confirm the diagnosis. If the radiograph is negative and there is a strong clinical suspicion, an isotope bone scan should be conducted (Fig. 7.4), which will reveal a focal area of increased uptake. Healing usually proceeds uneventfully if the patient has rest from the aggravating activity for six weeks. When there is no more pain when the aggravating movement is undertaken, and no local tenderness, activity can gradually be resumed. No cases of delayed union or nonunion of lower-rib stress fractures have been reported.

Strengthening of the serratus anterior by way of endurance exercises is an important component of the rehabilitation process.[17] Exercises should include protraction as well as

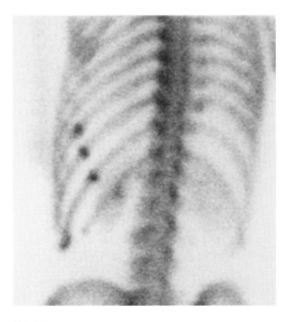

Fig. 7.4
An isotope bone scan that shows multiple stress fractures of the ribs.

flexion and abduction of the shoulder, in the coronal and scapular planes.

The pars interarticularis

The pars interarticularis is the narrow portion of bone that lies between the superior and inferior articular facets of the vertebral arch. Stress fracture of the pars is one of the more common stress fractures, and is especially common in sports that involve repeated hyperextension of the lower back. These stress fractures have a tendency to develop nonunion, because of the associated distraction forces.

Some confusion remains about use of the terms 'spondylolysis', 'pars defects' and 'stress fracture' with reference to the pars interarticularis. 'Spondylolysis' or 'pars defect' refers to existence of a defect in the pars interarticularis. This type of defect can be the result of nonunion of a stress fracture, or of a new fracture in which active bone remodeling occurs. The term 'stress fracture' of the pars should be confined to an active fracture in this area. The term 'spondylolisthesis' refers to complete bilateral defects in the pars interarticularis, including anterior displacement of one vertebra on another due to removal of the bony support from the vertebrae.

In spondylolysis, the bony defect may develop when the person is young, and it was in fact originally believed to be congenital.[34] However, the defect has never been shown to be present from birth: the youngest reported case is that of a child who was three-and-a-half months old. Few lesions of the pars have been detected in children who were less than five years old. Among children who were between five-and-a-half and six-and-a-half years of age, prevalence of spondylolysis jumps to about 5%,[35–39] and boys outnumber girls two to one.[38] In almost all cases, the children are completely pain free; in fact, in children who are less than ten years old it is unusual to see a symptomatic pars-interarticularis defect. After the age of ten, incidence of spondylolysis increases, especially among people who are involved in athletics.

Although most clinicians now believe that spondylolysis is acquired, in many cases fibrous union occurs; the defect becomes chronic, and there is evidence of neither bone remodeling nor healing.

Wiltse *et al.*[40] note that all but one of fourteen adolescents who had spondylolysis were engaged in vigorous sports at the time of the onset of their back pain. Hoshina[41] subjected the spine of 677 male secondary-school athletes to radiographic examination, and found that spondylolytic neural arches were present in more than 20% of the subjects. He notes that about 25% of the athletes who had spondylolysis had back pain, in contrast to only about 15% of the athletes who had intact neural arches. He also draws attention to the high incidence of associated anomalies, such as spina bifida and partial sacralization of the lumbar spine.

By adulthood, incidence of pars defects that are detectable by way of standard radiographic techniques is between 5% and 10%.[36,37] Spondylolysis has been reported in up to 30% of weightlifters between eighteen and twenty-four years of age who experienced back pain.[42] Ferguson *et al.*[43] report that half the interior linemen in one American Football team complained of back pain, and that of these, half had spondylolysis.

It is noted that in the American population, incidence of spondyloysis is higher in Whites than in Blacks, and higher in males than in females.[44] The Inuit population is noted to have one of the highest incidences of spondylolysis: as high as 50%.[45]

A definite familial tendency exists in development of pars interarticularis defects, especially in the case of defects that occur in the earlier years of life as opposed to ones that are acquired by adolescents who are involved in athletics. Rossi[42] found that of general-population cases, 30% of the people had a family history of either spondylolysis or

spondylolisthesis, whereas in the athlete population the familiarity was much less. Ciullo and Jackson[37] note that compared with the nonathletic population, there is a four-fold higher incidence of spondylolysis among gymnasts. There seems to be an increased incidence in association with spina-bifida occulta (Micheli, personal communication).

Although participation in sports increases the risk of developing spondylolysis, the risk varies from sport to sport. Incidence of spondylolysis among athletes in selected sports[42] is set out in Table 7.1.

Alexander[36] has identified three predominant movements and their associated sports that increase risk of spondylolysis. The sports are the ones in which the spine is loaded axially (weightlifting, and powerlifting), the ones in which there is a large component of rotation in the transverse plane (squash, racketball, tennis, baseball, and golf), and the ones in which the spine is either arched or extended (skiing, tennis, badminton, American Football, volleyball, basketball, rowing, gymnastics, cricket fast bowling, swimming, and diving).

Shear forces that act on the lumbar vertebrae increase when lumbar extension and, to a much lesser extent, flexion is undertaken. As the shear forces increase, pressure is transmitted from the facet joints to the pars interarticularis. Also,

Table 7.1 Incidence of spondylolysis in selected sports and the general population

Sport	Incidence (%)
Diving	63.3
Weightlifting	36.2
Wrestling	33.0
Gymnastics	32.0
Track and field	22.5
The general population	5.0

(Source: Adapted and reproduced, with permission, from Rossi F. Spondylolysis, spondylolisthesis and sports. Journal of Sports Medicine and Physical Fitness *1988; 18 (4): 317–340.)*

because the pars is small, it is predictably each vertebra's weakest anatomic link. Repetitive extension; flexion; hyperextension, including torsion,[41] and cyclic loading of the lumbar spine increase the shear forces across the facet and pars. Dissipation of loading forces through contraction of muscles may be reduced when the fatigue that is associated with repetitive activity occurs, and the result is that greater load is transmitted to the bone.[34] Although with marginal blood supply the bone undergoes remodeling, the rate of new-bone formation often lags behind that of bony resorption, especially if the lesion is asymptomatic and sport activity continues, whereby the result is a stress fracture.

Although pars defects are most commonly seen at L5, they are also found at L4 and L3. The athlete who has a pars stress fracture will usually complain of localized, unilateral low-back pain of insidious onset that is exacerbated by extension and/or rotation maneuvers. The pain is usually described as a chronic dull ache. The pain is often insufficient for preventing the athlete from continuing his or her activity.

When the patient is examined, he or she may have decreased lumbar flexibility, and hamstring tightness. If a one-leg hyperextension test is positive (Fig. 7.5), the diagnosis is strongly suggested.[46] There may be some localized tenderness close to the mid-line, at the appropriate level.

Once there is clinical suspicion of stress fracture of the pars, a radiographic examination should be conducted. X-rays of the lumbar spine should include an anteroposterior, a lateral, and an oblique view. The oblique view shows the typical 'scotty dog' outline (Fig. 7.6 a). A radiolucent collar on the 'scotty dog' represents a defect of the pars interarticularis (Fig. 7.6 b). If the collar is sclerotic, it probably represents a healing pars fracture. If a pars defect is present, there may be either an old fracture that has healed by a fibrous union or an active recent fracture. However, an acute stress fracture of relatively recent onset will usually fail to show any abnormality on plain radiograph.

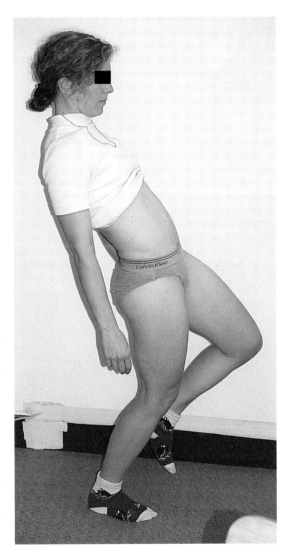

Fig. 7.5
A one-legged hyperextension test for stress fracture of the pars interarticularis.

For patients whose clinical presentation is consistent with stress fracture of the pars but who have a normal radiograph, a bone scan, or preferably a single photon emission computed tomography (SPECT) scan, should be conducted. A SPECT scan is preferred to a normal technetium scan, because of its increased sensitivity. On a SPECT scan (Fig. 7.7), presence

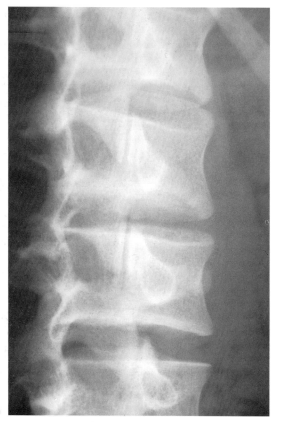

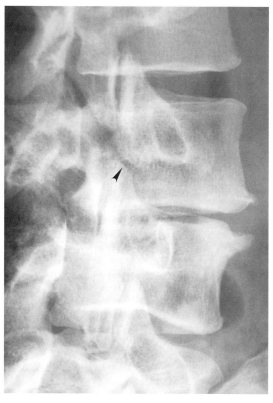

Fig. 7.6

a An oblique radiograph of the lumbar spine that shows the normal 'scotty dog' appearance; **b** A pars defect that shows a break in the continuity of the neck of the 'scotty dog'.

of a focal area of increased uptake confirms presence of an active stress fracture.

If, on the oblique radiograph, a pars defect is present that is associated with the typical clinical picture of a pars stress fracture, many clinicians would consider this to be sufficient for making the diagnosis. We consider that a SPECT scan is necessary in order to confirm presence of an active fracture rather than of an old fracture that includes fibrous union.

If more delineation of the lesion is required, a CT scan (Fig. 7.8) should be conducted in order to determine the lesion's site and extent. Congeni *et al.*[47] followed a group of 40 patients who had

low-back pain, who had a normal plain radiograph, and who had a positive SPECT scan, and conducted CT scans ten weeks after diagnosis following a rehabilitation program. The CT appearances were divided into three groups. Eighteen of the subjects (45%) had a chronic, nonhealed fracture; sixteen (40%) had an acute fracture in various stages of healing; and in six (15%), no complete fracture was noted. Several of the lastmentioned subjects showed an increased uptake on SPECT but no bony disruption. A patient who presents with an appropriate clinical picture, a positive SPECT scan, and a normal CT scan should be considered

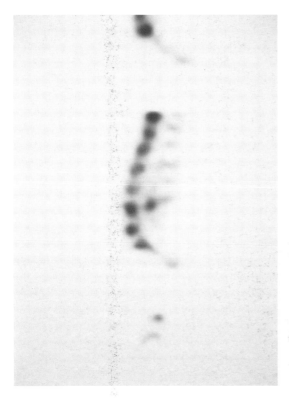

Fig. 7.7
A SPECT scan that shows an area of increased uptake that indicates an active stress fracture of the pars interarticularis.

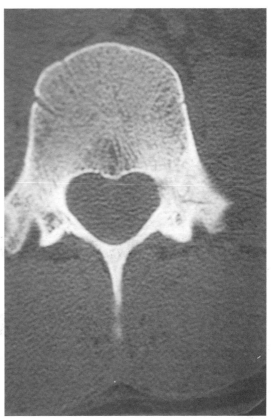

Fig. 7.8
A CT scan of a stress fracture of the pars interarticularis.

to have an early stress fracture, and should be treated aggressively. This group of patients may have the best chance of healing (Micheli, personal communication).

Considerable variation exists in the recommended treatment for pars stress fractures. Almost all clinicians agree it is necessary to restrict the athletic activity that is responsible for the pain, to stretch the hamstring and gluteal muscles, and to strengthen the abdominal and back extensor muscles as soon as the exercises can be undertaken pain free. However, it is debatable whether or not antilordotic bracing should be used.

Micheli *et al.*[48] studied seventy-five adolescent athletes for whom 'spondylolysis' had been diagnosed by way of a positive bone scan, and who were placed in a modified Boston antilordotic brace (Fig. 7.9) for twenty-three hours per day for three to six months. Eighty-eight percent of the athletes improved and returned to activity. However, of them, only 32% healed by way of a bony union. In another study that involved the same group of sixty-seven patients who had symptomatic spondylolysis, 78% of the patients had either an excellent or a good result, no pain, and return to full activity; 13% continued to have mild symptoms; and six (9%) subsequently required fusion *in situ*. Only twelve (18%) showed radiographic evidence that their pars defect/s had healed.

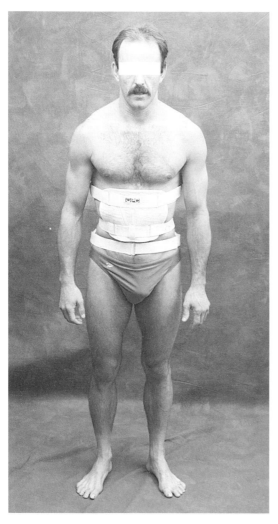

Fig. 7.9
A Boston antilordotic brace.

In two recent Japanese studies, by Morita *et al.*[52] and Katoh *et al.*[53] healing at various stages of spondylolysis was compared. The researchers[52,53] classified pars defects into three stages: early, progressive, and terminal. The early stage was characterized by either focal bony absorption or a hairline defect on radiographic appearance. In the progressive stage, the defect was wide, and small fragments were present. Sclerotic change indicated the terminal stage of development.

In Morita *et al.*'s study,[52] the researchers retrospectively reviewed the progress of pars defects at 193 levels in 185 patients who completed their treatment regimen, which at first consisted of discontinuing their sport and wear-ing a conventional lumbar corset for three to six months. Follow-up radiographs were taken at four-week intervals. Once the defect had united, the patients followed a rehabilitation protocol while wearing a special lumbosacral support that enabled them to have full flexion but that restricted extension of the lumbar spine. Overall, 37.9% of all the pars defects had apparent radio-logic healing. Union was achieved in 73% of the early-stage defects, in 39% of the progressive-stage defects, and in none of the terminal-stage defects. The researchers also found that incidence of union of unilateral defects was significantly higher than incidence of union of bilateral defects, and found no differences in the rates of healing for same-stage defects in three age groups: less than thirteen years of age, thirteen to fifteen years of age, and fifteen to eighteen years of age.

In Katoh *et al.*'s study,[53] similar results were shown for the three stages of spondylolysis. An improved rate of union was also shown in defects at L4, compared with those at L5, and in lesions that were closer to the vertebral body.

From these studies, it would seem that it is the defect's stage and site, not the type of treatment, that determines the bony defect's healing. It is therefore important that an early diagnosis be made and that a treatment program be commenced that consists of rest from sport, as well as rehabilitation.

Other clinicians recommend there be activity restriction without bracing. Some recommend complete bed rest until the symptoms have subsided,[49] whereas others recommend there be an active rest period during which the athlete participates in activities that do not aggravate the symptoms.[34,37,38,40,42,50,51] Considerable variation exists as to the time scale for activity restriction.

We believe there should not be a set period of time, but that the patient should at first undergo a rehabilitation program that involves pain-free progressive exercises that do not include the aggravating activity: lumbar extension and/or rotation. When the patient can undertake the aggravating maneuvers pain free, and there is no local tenderness, he or she should gradually and progressively resume the aggravating activity over a period of four to six weeks, using pain as a guide.

Saal[54] suggests that the rehabilitation program be based on thorough patient-examination findings and an understanding of the problem's pathophysiology. Upper extremity, lower extremity, and trunk flexibility and strength, as well as alignment of the spine and lower extremities, must be assessed. Muscles that are especially important are the iliopsoas, quadriceps, hamstrings, abdominals, latissimus dorsi, erector spinae, tensor fascia lata, hip rotators, and hip extensors.

The abdominal wall muscles, especially the internal oblique and transverse abdominus muscles as well as the latissimus dorsi, help stabilize the lumbar spine through their attachments to the thoracolumbar fascia.[55,56] The lumbar paraspinal muscles, especially the multifidus, are also important in prevention of shear forces in the lumbar spine.[54,55,57,58] The abdominal muscles are also important for positioning the pelvis in order to receive trunk forces.[59]

Exercise programs for stabilizing the lumbar spine have been developed as a result of this understanding of muscle forces.[58] Appropriate spinal-stabilization exercise programs are described by a number of researchers.[54,57,60–62] Electrical stimulation should be considered for young patients who remain symptomatic after treatment, and for skeletally mature people who have a higher rate of persistent symptoms (see Chapter 5).

Some pars injuries may heal with elongation of the pars. This elongation may result in disruption of the facet's normal articulation with

Table 7.2 Percentage of slip

Grade	Slip (%)
1	0–25
2	25–50
3	50–70
4	> 75

its adjacent facet, and in overload of the entire segment, thereby increasing the risk of degenerative change. The patient requires monitoring and good back care.

A unilateral pars defect may result in increasing stress to the contralateral pars, which results in bilateral spondylolysis. Spondylolisthesis may occur in the presence of a bilateral pars defect (Fig. 7.10). Spondylolisthesis that is secondary to stress fracture of the pars tends to occur during the adolescent years, and is rarely seen once skeletal maturity has been reached. In the older patient, spondylolisthesis is usually associated with degenerative change.

The percentage of slip is graded as set out in Table 7.2.

Most clinicians would consider that adolescent athletes who have a Grade 1 slip are able to participate in sports without restriction, and that the ones who have a Grade 2 slip are able to participate in sports that are low risk with reference to back injury. These patients must be followed closely for any evidence of progression. For adolescents who have a Grade 3 or a Grade 4 slippage, a surgical stabilization procedure should be conducted

In a study in which a group of sixty-four children and adolescents were studied who were between six and twenty years of age and who had spondylolisthesis at L5 over an average of 4.8 years, none of the patients had cause to stop training. Eight patients who had a Stage 2 and two patients who had a Stage 3 spondylolisthesis were included in the study. Only ten of the athletes had progression (an increase in displacement of >10%) in their spondylolisthesis. This rate is comparable to that

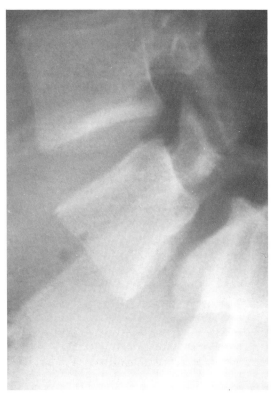

Fig. 7.10
Bilateral pars defects, with Grade 1 spondylolisthesis.

found in other studies,[63–65] in which the subjects did not play a sport.

TREATMENT SUMMARY

A patient for whom spondylolysis is clinically suspected should have an oblique radiograph. If the radiograph reveals either a defect or sclerosis, the next step should be a SPECT scan. If the SPECT scan reveals an active fracture, it is recommended that the patient cease the aggravating activity, wear a lumbar corset and, when he or she is pain free when active movements are undertaken, commence a rehabilitation program in which the emphasis is on spinal stabilization.

The lumbar spine: other stress fractures

Other lumbar-spine stress fractures that are reported in the literature include a pedicle fracture in a ballet dancer,[66] laminar fractures in a jogger,[67] and laminar and pars fractures in a very active child, caused by lifting heavy objects and scrubbing floors.[68]

Fehlandt and Micheli[66] describe the case of a ballerina who had a stress fracture of the fourth lumbar inferior articular facet. The ballerina was thirty-six years old, had twenty eight years' dance training, and was in her eighteenth year of professional dancing. She complained of left lower-back pain that had developed insidiously during a month of vigorous performing and rehearsing. The pain was exacerbated by a dance that involved repetitive hyperextension and rotation of the spine, whereby the spine was placed in a hyperextended position, draped over another dancer's shoulder. When the ballerina was examined, she had left-lumbar paravertebral muscle spasm and increased pain when hyperextension and left-lateral flexion were undertaken. Lumbar-spine radiographs revealed mild degenerative changes of the lower-lumbar facet joints, sclerosis of the pars interarticularis, and neither spondylolysis nor spondylolisthesis. A SPECT scan revealed increased tracer uptake in the L4 posterior elements, and a CT scan showed pars interarticularis sclerosis, and irregularity in the dorsal contour of the left L4 inferior facet.

Although the ballerina was at first diagnosed as having a stress fracture of the pars interarticularis, persistence of her symptoms and of the irregularity of the dorsal contour of the left L4 inferior articular facet suggested there was a stress fracture of the facet joint. Anesthetic injected into the facet joint produced temporary pain relief. Sixteen months after the earlier presentation, the left L4 inferior articular facet was surgically explored. The facet's entire margin had osteophytic lipping. At the inferolateral aspect of the left L4 inferior articular facet, an oblique fracture through the facet was identified, including nonunion of the fracture fragment. The loose fragment was excised. Two months after surgery, the ballerina resumed dancing, without restrictions.

We have seen one facet joint stress fracture, as shown in Fig. 7.11.

The sacrum

A few reports have been published of stress fracture of the sacrum among athletes. Bottomley[69] reports the case of a 28-year-old female 10,000 meter runner who presented with a 10-day history of insidious-onset pain in the right buttock. When the patient was examined, there was acute and very localized tenderness in the upper outer quadrant of the right buttock. A plain radiograph of the lumbar spine and pelvis revealed no significant abnormality. An isotope bone scan conducted eighteen days after the pain's onset showed slightly increased uptake at the lower end of the right sacro-iliac joint, on the sacral side. Diagnosis of sacro-iliac strain was made, and an injection of corticosteroid and local anesthetic was given. The patient was restricted to water running for two weeks. Any attempt at running exacerbated the pain. Two weeks later, the patient competed, and performed well below her normal standard. It was noted at the time that her percentage body fat was only 9 percent, and subsequent measurement of bone-mineral density showed marked reduction in bone density. This was believed to be secondary to prolonged amenorrhea. It was postulated that a leg-length discrepancy of approximately half an inch may have been another significant factor in the etiology of the problem.

Holtzhausen and Noakes[70] report two cases of stress fracture of the sacrum. In the first case, a 42-year-old male marathon runner developed severe pain in the right buttock at the 18 kilometer point of a 21 kilometer foot race.

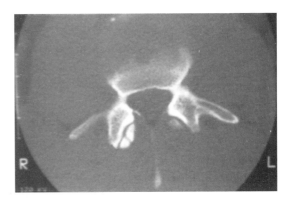

Fig. 7.11
CT-scan appearance of a stress fracture of the lumbar facet joint.

Although the pain was subsequently relieved when the patient had a week of rest, it recurred when he attempted to run distances greater than 8 kilometers. In the year before the injury occurred, the patient had completed fourteen marathon and six ultramarathon races for a total of more than 1300 kilometers' worth of competition running. He had also progressively increased his training mileage and speed. When he was clinically examined, some tenderness to palpation was found over the region of the right sacro-iliac joint. Radiographs of the pelvis and lumbar spine revealed no bony abnormalities. An isotope bone scan showed increased uptake in the area of the right sacral ala, and this was more diffuse than focal.

In the second case, a 35-year-old, male, elite distance runner developed acute debilitating pain in the left buttock while competing in a 21 kilometer race. He described the onset of pain at the 18 kilometer point as being a sudden 'give' in his left hip, 'as though the gluteal muscles had been torn'. For some months before the injury occurred, he had increased his weekly training mileage from 80 to 180 kilometers. When he was clinically examined, a well-localized area of tenderness was found over the left sacro-iliac joint, and there was also limited hip extension.

An isotope bone scan conducted three weeks after the injury's onset revealed a sharply demarcated oval-shaped area of increased bony activity in the region of the left sacral ala, an appearance similar to that shown in Fig. 7.12. The patient was advised to engage in non-weightbearing activities until the pain disappeared. Seven weeks after the injury occurred, he resumed jogging. The researchers state that the sacral alae are subjected to repeated cyclical loading when vigorous weightbearing exercise is undertaken, whereby the body's weight that is distributed from the vertebral column via the sacral ala to the lower limbs is counteracted by a ground-reaction force at the acetabulum and the symphysis pubis. These lines of force form a complete ring around the pelvic ring, which includes the sacral alae.

Haasbeek and Green[71] present two more cases that involved teenage female athletes. In the first

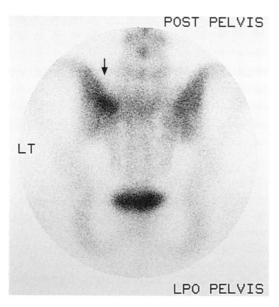

POST PELVIS

LT

LPO PELVIS

Fig. 7.12
An isotope bone scan image of a stress fracture of the sacrum.

case, a fifteen-year-old girl presented with a one-year history of low-back pain that had worsened over the preceding two weeks. The pain was localized over the area of the right sacro-iliac joint, but spread laterally to the wing of the ilium, and distally into the upper half of the buttock. Radiographs of the lumbosacral spine and pelvis were unremarkable. Isotope bone scans revealed increased uptake in the area of the right sacro-iliac joint. In a SPECT scan, the increased uptake was localized to the anterior aspect of the sacrum, just medial to the sacro-iliac joint. A CT scan showed irregularity and sclerosis over the superior aspect of the right sacral ala that correlated with the geographic location of the bone scan abnormalities. The patient was treated by having seven weeks of crutch walking, and non-weightbearing on the right side. She was subsequently rehabilitated by way of undertaking a progressive program of strengthening exercises, and returned to full activity with no symptom recurrence.

In the second case, a sixteen-year-old female runner had a two-week history of low-back pain. She had been running six to seven miles per day for several years, and had had no change in her training schedule. Her pain was present before, during, and after running, but was worse during and immediately after each run. She also noted she had increased pain when running downhill. When she was examined, the pain was localized to the right side of the lumbosacral region, and spread toward the wing of the ilium and into the cephalad portion of the right buttock. Hyperextension reproduced the patient's pain. Radiographs of the lumbosacral spine and pelvis were negative. An isotope bone scan revealed increased uptake over the right anterior sacrum, and this was especially well visualized on SPECT images. A CT scan confirmed a stress fracture of the right anterior sacral ala. Treatment consisted of partial weightbearing on the right side, including use of crutches, for a period of eight weeks.

Czarnecki *et al.*[72] describe a case of stress fractures of the body of the sacrum. They comment that the plain radiography findings may be either normal or easily overlooked because of either overlying bowel gas or osteopenia. Findings by way of isotope bone scan may show an H-shaped or butterfly-shaped pattern of uptake that is consistent with bilateral vertical fractures, and a single transverse fracture that involves the sacral ala. CT findings typically show a sclerotic vertical fracture, parallel to the sacro-iliac joint. Some fractures may be bilateral, and have a transverse component.

Atwell and Jackson[73] report two cases of male runners who developed pain in the gluteal area. In both cases, a SPECT scan revealed increased uptake. Although in one case stress fracture was confirmed by way of MRI (there was a decreased marrow signal in the anterolateral sacrum), in the other case an MRI taken before the SPECT scan was conducted failed to show any abnormality. Both patients returned to running, at three and five weeks, respectively.

McFarland and Giangarra[74] report three cases of sacral stress fracture in female athletes, all of whom presented with low-back and/or buttock pain. Plain-radiograph films were normal, and the diagnosis was confirmed by way of isotope bone scan. The fractures healed uneventfully when the patients rested.

Eller *et al.*[75] report three cases of sacral stress fracture in female long-distance runners, all of whom presented with unilateral sacro-iliac pain. MRI revealed presence of bone-marrow edema, and a linear fracture line. The researchers believed that the MRI enabled them to differentiate between sacral stress fracture and problems of the sacro-iliac joint, as well as between stress reaction and stress fracture. Each of the patients in the series was amenorrheic and had subnormal bone density.

Gerrard and Doyle[76] describe the case of a 35-year-old female long-distance runner who experienced lower-back and buttock pain during a track workout that comprised 200 meter repetitions. When she was examined, she had focal tenderness over the right sacro-iliac region, and it was possible to reproduce her pain by way of one-leg standing and hopping. A SPECT scan revealed a focal area of intense uptake in the lower part of the anterior surface of the right sacral wing. A CT scan showed a fine fracture line, including surrounding reactive sclerosis. The patient ceased running for one month, then gradually returned to full activity. The researchers state that compared with road running, the varied biomechanics of 200 meter track running were the likely origin of the lumbosacral pain.

SUMMARY

- Patients who have a stress fracture of the first rib present with gradual onset of shoulder pain and medial scapular pain, including local tenderness.
- Stress fractures of the lower ribs are common among golfers and rowers, and should not be confused with an intercostal muscle strain.
- Pars-interarticularis stress fractures occur when activities are undertaken that involve repeated hyperextension.
- It is important to differentiate between an active stress fracture, which shows increased uptake on a SPECT scan, and an old pars defect, in which fibrous union has occurred.
- We advocate a rehabilitation program that at first involves pain-free exercises, followed by progression to gradual resumption of the aggravating activity.
- Some clinicians recommend a brace be used in order to limit extension.
- Stress fractures of the sacrum have been described among distance runners.

References

1. Keating TM. Stress fracture of the sternum in a wrestler. *American Journal of Sports Medicine* 1987; 15: 92–93.

2. Barbaix EJ. Stress fracture of the sternum in a golf player. *International Journal of Sports Medicine* 1996; 17: 303–304.

3. Robertsen K, Kristensen O, Vejen L. Manubrium sterni stress fracture: an unusual complication of non-contact sport. *British Journal of Sports Medicine* 1996; 30 (2): 176–177.

4. Curran JP, Kelly DA. Stress fracture of the first rib. *American Journal of Orthopedic Surgery* 1966; 8: 16–18.

5. Gurtler R, Pavlov H, Torg JS. Stress fracture of the ipsilateral first rib in a pitcher. *American Journal of Sports Medicine* 1985; 13: 277–279.

6. Lankenner PAJ, Micheli LJ. Stress fracture of the first rib: a case report. *Journal of Bone and Joint Surgery* 1985; 67A: 159–160.

7. Rademaker M, Redmond AD, Barker PV. Stress fracture of the first rib. *Thorax* 1983; 38: 312–313.

8. Sacchetti AD, Beswick DR, Morse SD. Rebound rib: stress induced first rib fracture. *Annals of Emergency Medicine* 1983; 12: 177–179.

9. Mintz AC, Albano A, Reisdorff EJ, Choe KA, Lillegard W. Stress fracture of the first rib from serratus anterior tension: an unusual mechanism of injury. *Annals of Emergency Medicine* 1990; 19 (4): 411–414.

10. Crichton KJ, Bradshaw CJ, Brown JM, Hartwright D. Stress fracture of the first rib in ballet dancers. (In preparation.)

11. Ochi M, Sasashige Y, Murakami T, Ikuta Y. Brachial plexus palsy secondary to stress fracture of the first rib: case report. *Journal of Trauma* 1994; 36 (1): 128–130.

12. Blichert-Toft M. Fatigue fracture of the first rib. *Acta Chirurgia Scandanavica* 1968; 135: 675–678.

13. Barrett GR, Shelton WR, Miles JW. First rib fractures in football players: a case report and literature review. *American Journal of Sports Medicine* 1988; 16: 674–676.

14. Derbes VJ, Harran T. Rib fracture from muscular effort with particular reference to cough. *Surgery* 1954; 35: 294–321.

15. Rassad S. Golfer's fractures of the ribs: report of three cases. *American Journal of Roentgenology, Radiotherapy and Nuclear Medicine* 1974; 120: 901–903.

16. Holden DL, Jackson DW. Stress fracture of the ribs in female rowers. *American Journal of Sports Medicine* 1985; 13: 342–348.

17. Lord MJ, Carson WG. Multiple rib stress fractures: a golfer overdoes it – case report. *Physician and Sportsmedicine* 1993; 21 (5): 80–91.

18. Hsu CY, Lin HC, Kao WY, Lin WY, Wan SJ. Stress fracture of the ribs in amateur golfers diagnosed by Tc-99m MDP scintigraphy. *Kao Hsuing I Hsueh Ko Hsueh Tsa Chih* 1993; 9 (6): 381–384.

19. Orava S, Kallinen M, Aito H, Aln M. Stress fracture of the ribs in golfers: a report of five cases. *Scandinavian Journal of Medicine and Science in Sports* 1994; 4 (2): 155–158.

20. Read MTF. Case report – stress fracture of the rib in a golfer. *British Journal of Sports Medicine* 1994; 28 (3): 206–207.

21. Lin HC, Chou CS, Hsu TC. Stress fractures of the ribs in amateur golf players. *Chung Hua I Hsueh Tsa Chih (Taipei)* 1994; 54 (1): 33–37.

22. Lord MJ, Ha KI, Song KS. Stress fractures of the ribs in golfers. *American Journal of Sports Medicine* 1996; 24 (1): 118–122.

23. Goyal M, Kenney AJ, Hanelin LG. Golfer's rib stress fracture (Duffer's fracture): scintigraphic appearance. *Clinical Nuclear Medicine* 1997; 22 (7): 503–504.

24. McKenzie DC. Stress fracture of the rib in an elite oarsman. *International Journal of Sports Medicine* 1989; 10: 220–222.

25. Brukner P, Khan K. Stress fracture of the posterior aspect of the ribs in a rower: case report. *Clinical Journal of Sport Medicine* 1996; 6 (3): 204–206.

26. Christiansen E, Kanstrup IL. Increased risk of stress fractures of the ribs in elite rowers. *Scandinavian Journal of Medicine and Science in Sports* 1997; 7 (1): 49–52.

27. Molvaer OI. Stress fracture in ribs due to river paddling. *Tidsskrift for den Norske Laegeforening* 1976; 96 (3): 149–150, 153.

28. Orava S, Jakkola L, Kujala UM. Stress fracture of the seventh rib in a squash player. *Scandinavian Journal of Medicine and Science in Sports* 1991; 1: 247–248.

29. Taimela S, Kujala UN, Orava S. Two consecutive rib stress fractures in a female competitive swimmer. *Clinical Journal of Sport Medicine* 1995; 5 (4): 254–257.

30. Seilin J. Fracture of the 11th rib by muscular action: résumé of reported cases. *Med. Rec.* 1917; 91: 281–283.

31. Tunis JP. Rib fracture from muscular action with 40 collected cases. *University Medical Magazine* 1890; 3: 57–65.

32. Oechsli WR. Rib fractures from cough. *Journal of Thoracic Surgery* 1936; 5: 530–534.

33. Satou S, Konisi N. The mechanism of fatigue fracture of the ribs. *Journal of the Japanese Orthopaedic Association* 1991; 65: 708–719.

34. Letts M, Smallman T, Afanasiev R, Gouw G. Fracture of the pars interarticularis in adolescent athletes: a clinical–biomechanical analysis. *Journal of Pediatric Orthopedics* 1986; 6 (1): 40–46.

35 Frederikson B, Baker D, McHolick WJ, Yuan HA, Lubicky JP. The natural history of spondylolysis and spondylolysthesis. *Journal of Bone and Joint Surgery* 1984; 66-A: 699–707.

36 Alexander MJL. Biomechanical aspects of lumbar spine in athletes. *Canadian Journal of Applied Sports Sciences* 1985; 10: 1–10.

37 Ciullo JV, Jackson DW. Pars interarticularis stress reaction, spondylolysis and spondylolisthesis in gymnasts. *Clinics in Sports Medicine* 1985; 4: 95–110.

38 Brigham CD, Schafer MF. Low back pain in athletes. *Advances in Sports Medicine and Fitness* 1988; 1: 145–182.

39 Weir MR, Smith DS. Stress reaction of the pars interarticularis leading to spondylolysis: a cause of adolescent low back pain. *Journal of Adolescent Health Care* 1989; 10 (6): 573–577.

40 Wiltse LL, Widell EHJ, Jackson DW. Fatigue fracture: the basic lesion in isthmic spondylolisthesis. *Journal of Bone and Joint Surgery* 1975; 57S: 17–22.

41 Hoshina H. Spondylolysis in athletes. *Physician and Sportsmedicine* 1980; 8 (9): 75–97.

42 Rossi F. Spondylolysis, spondylolisthesis and sports. *Journal of Sports Medicine and Physical Fitness* 1988; 18 (4): 317–340.

43 Ferguson RI, McMasters JH, Stanitski CC. Low back pain in college football linemen. *American Journal of Sports Medicine* 1974; 2: 63.

44 Roche MB, Rowe GG. The incidence of separate neural arch and coincident bone variations. *Journal of Bone and Joint Surgery* 1952; 34A: 491–494.

45 Stewart TD. The age incidence of neural arch defects in Alaska Natives, considered from the viewpoint of etiology. *Journal of Bone and Joint Surgery (Am)* 1953; 35: 937–950.

46 Keene JS. Low back pain in the athlete: from spondylogenic injury during recreation or competition. *Postgraduate Medicine* 1983; 74 (6): 209–217.

47 Congeni J, McCulloch J, Swanson K. Lumbar spondylolysis: a study of natural progression in athletes. *American Journal of Sports Medicine* 1997; 25 (2): 248–253.

48 Micheli MJ, Hall JE, Miller ME. Use of modified Boston brace for back injuries in athletes. *American Journal of Sports Medicine* 1980; 8 (5): 351–359.

49 Goldberg MJ. Gymnastics injuries. *Orthopedic Clinics of North America* 1980; 11: 717–723.

50 Jackson DW, Wiltes LL, Dingman RD, Hays M. Stress reactions involving the pars interarticularis in young athletes. *American Journal of Sports Medicine* 1981; 9: 304–312.

51 Flemming JE. Spondylolysis and spondylolysthesis in the athlete. In: Hochschuler SH, ed. *The Spine in Sports*. Philadelphia: Hanley and Belfus, 1990: 101–107.

52 Morita T, Ikata T, Katoh S, Miyake R. Lumbar spondylolysis in children and adolescents. *Journal of Bone and Joint Surgery* 1995; 77-B (4): 620–625.

53 Katoh S, Ikata T, Fujii K. Factors influencing nonunion of spondylolysis in children and adolescents. (Abstract.) *North American Spine Society: 12th Annual Meeting.* New York, 1997.

54 Saal JA. Rehabilitation of sports related lumbar spine injuries. *Physical Medicine and Rehabilitation: State of the Art Reviews* 1987; 1: 613–638.

55 Farfan HF, Osteria V, Lamy C. The mechanical etiology of spondylolysis and spondylolysthesis. *Clinical Orthopedics and Related Research* 1976; 117: 40–55.

56 Bogduk N, MacIntosh JE. The applied anatomy of the thoracolumbar fascia. *Spine* 1984; 9: 164–170.

57 Saal JA. Rehabilitation of football players with lumbar spine injury. *Physician and Sportsmedicine* 1988; 16: 117–125.

58 Weber MD, Woodall WR. Spondylogenic disorders in gymnasts. *Journal of Orthopaedic and Sports Physical Therapy* 1991; 14: 6–13.

59 Porterfield JA. The sacroiliac joint. In: Gould JA, Davies GJ, eds. *Orthopaedics and Sports Physical Therapy*. St Louis: CV Mosby Company, 1985: 550–558.

60 Gustavson R, Streeck R. *Training Therapy: Prophylaxis and Rehabilitation*. New York: Thieme Inc., 1985.

61 Saal JA, Saal JS. Nonoperative treatment of herniated lumbar intervertebral disc with radiculopathy. *Spine* 1989; 14: 431–437.

62 Morgan D. Concepts in functional training and postural stabilisation for the low-back-injured. *Topics in Acute Care Trauma and Rehabilitation* 1988; 2: 8–17.

63 McPhee IB, O'Brien JP, McCall IW, Park WM. Progression of lumbosacral spondylolisthesis. *Australian Radiology* 1981; 25: 91–94.

64 Blackburne BJS, Velikas EP. Spondylolysthesis in children and adolescents. *Journal of Bone and Joint Surgery (Br)* 1977; 59: 490–494.

65 Seitsalo S, Osterman K, Hyvarinen H *et al.* Progression of spondylolysthesis in children and adolescents: a long term followup of 272 patients. *Spine* 1991; 16: 417–421.

66 Fehlandt AF, Micheli MJ. Lumbar facet stress fracture in a ballet dancer. *Spine* 1993; 18 (16): 2537–2539.

67 Abel MA. Jogger's fractures and other stress fractures on the lumbar sacral spine. *Skeletal Radiology* 1985; 13: 221–227.

[68] Daffner RH. Stress fractures: current concepts. *Skeletal Radiology* 1978; 2: 221–229.

[69] Bottomley MB. Sacral stress fracture in a runner. *British Journal of Sports Medicine* 1990; 24 (4): 243–244.

[70] Holtzhausen L, Noakes TD. Stress fracture of the sacrum in two distance runners. *Clinical Journal of Sport Medicine* 1992; 2: 139–142.

[71] Haasbeek JF, Green NE. Adolescent stress fractures of the sacrum: two case reports. *Journal of Pedriatric Orthopaedics* 1994; 14: 336–338.

[72] Czarnecki DJ, Till EW, Minikel JL. Unique sacral stress fracture in a runner. (Letter.) *American Journal of Radiology* 1988; 151: 1255.

[73] Atwell EA, Jackson DW. Stress fractures of the sacrum in runners: two case reports. *American Journal of Sports Medicine* 1991; 19: 531–533.

[74] McFarland EG, Giangarra C. Sacral stress fractures in athletes. *Clinical Orthopedics* 1996; 329: 240–243.

[75] Eller DJ, Katz DS, Bergman AG, Fredericson M, Beaulieu CF. Sacral stress fractures in long-distance runners. *Clinical Journal of Sport Medicine* 1997; 7: 222–225.

[76] Gerrard DF, Doyle TCA. Lumbosacral pain in an athlete: an unusual site for stress fracture. *Clinical Journal of Sport Medicine* 1998; 8: 59–61.

Chapter 8

Stress fractures of the pelvis and thigh

Stress fractures in this region are reasonably common, especially among distance runners. Stress fracture of the neck of the femur is one of the small group of stress fractures for which specific treatment is required.

The pubic ramus

Noakes *et al.*[1] describe five cases of radiographically proven stress fracture of the pubic ramus among distance runners, three of whom were elite female marathoners. In another two cases, in which radiography failed to support the clinical diagnosis, evidence of stress fracture was revealed by way of isotope bone scan. Although another five cases had identically the same clinical presentation, the diagnosis was not confirmed radiologically, and an isotope bone scan was not conducted.

The researchers stated that a diagnosis of pubic ramus stress fracture can confidently be made, even when radiographic evidence is absent, when the following three features are present in a long-distance runner who presents with groin pain.

1. Activity causes such severe discomfort in the groin that running is impossible.
2. The athlete develops discomfort in the groin when standing unsupported on the leg that corresponds to the injured side.
3. Deep palpation reveals extreme, exquisite, nauseating tenderness that is localized to the pubic ramus, not to the overlying soft tissues.

Stress fractures of the pubic ramus (Fig. 8.1) seem to occur almost exclusively in female long-distance runners who have a reduced bone-mineral density that is secondary to prolonged periods of menstrual irregularity, and possibly to an eating disorder.

These stress fractures seem to heal without complication if the aggravating activity is avoided for a period of eight to twelve weeks. Naturally, it is necessary to pay attention to the precipitating factors.

The femoral neck

Stress fracture of the femoral neck is a stress fracture for which early recognition is required in order to prevent potentially serious complications. This type of fracture was first described by Earnst,[2] who presented thirteen cases. Devas[3] subsequently described twenty-five cases, and Blickenstaff and Morris[4] thirty-six cases. Fullerton and Snowdy[5] categorized the types of fracture, and Fullerton[6] has written an excellent review of the topic.

There are two distinct types of femoral stress fracture (Fig. 8.2), as follows.

1. Fractures on the superior aspect of the neck, known as the tension or distraction side, which are mainly seen in older patients
2. Fractures on the inferior aspect of the neck, known as the compression side, which are seen in younger patients

For both sites, a spectrum of changes is shown (Fig. 8.3), as follows.

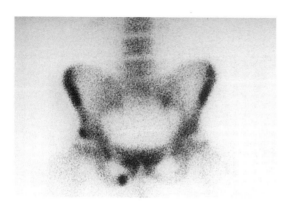

Fig. 8.1
An isotope bone scan of a stress fracture of the pubic ramus.

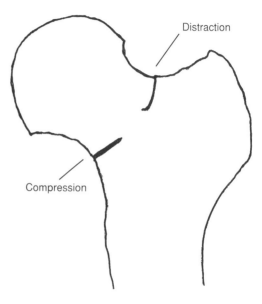

Fig. 8.2
The sites of femoral neck stress fractures.

- Stage 1: For this stage, there is a normal radiograph, and a positive isotope bone scan.
- Stage 2: The next stage is manifest with either endosteal or periosteal callus, without a fracture.
- Stage 3: A cortical crack, without displacement, follows.
- Stage 4: The final stages are widening of the cortical crack, followed by displacement.[6]

The patient usually presents with a history of anterior hip or groin pain that is aggravated by exercise. Night pain is occasionally present. The physical examination may reveal pain and restriction at the end range of passive hip movement. There is occasionally tenderness to deep palpation over the femoral neck.

For the athlete who has exercise-related groin or hip pain, a plain radiograph should be taken. However, in a study by Fullerton and Snowdy,[5] radiographs that were taken soon after the symptoms began were positive in fewer than 20% of cases of femoral neck stress fracture. An isotope bone scan should be conducted if there is any clinical suspicion of stress fracture. Although there have occasionally been cases of a negative bone scan for athletes who subsequently developed radiographic evidence of stress fracture,[7,8] most series indicate that isotope bone scan is the most discriminating diagnostic test. In most cases, repeat radiographs will become positive in one or two weeks.[9]

Shin *et al.*[10] evaluated the accuracy of MRI (Fig. 8.4) for nineteen military recruits who presented with twenty-two 'stress fractures', and who had hip pain, negative radiographs, and a positive isotope bone scan. Each patient underwent MRI, then had a follow-up radiograph at six weeks, in order to verify the diagnosis of stress fracture. In five of the twenty-two studies, diagnosis of femoral stress fracture was excluded by way of the MRI findings, and the patients were allowed to return early to full military duty. The diagnoses included a synovial pit, an iliopsoas tear, bilateral iliopsoas tendonitis, and obturator externus tendonitis. For one patient, not only was a femoral neck stress fracture excluded; a unicameral bone cyst was identified as being present. For another patient, the MRI findings were consistent with early avascular necrosis of the femoral head. For the cases in which stress fractures were suspected, MRI revealed bone changes before the radiographs identified them.

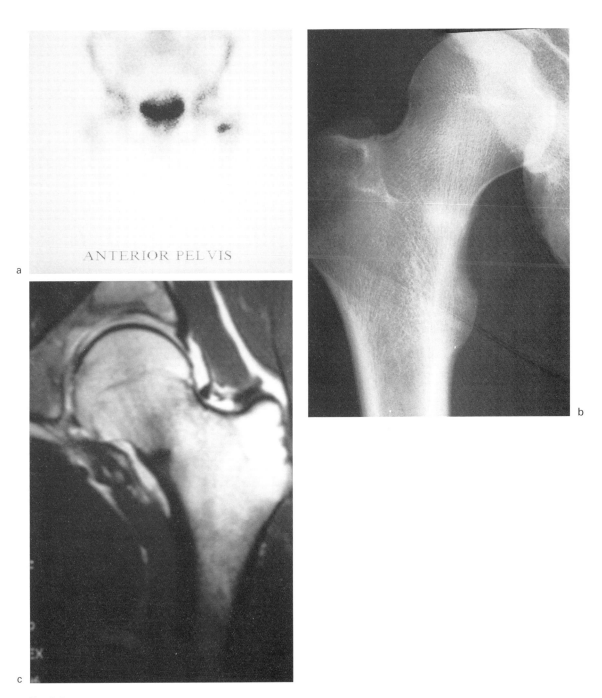

Fig. 8.3

The first three stages of femoral-neck stress fracture: **a** A normal radiograph, and a positive isotope bone scan (shown); **b** periosteal callus, with no fracture line; **c** MRI showing a cortical crack, without displacement.

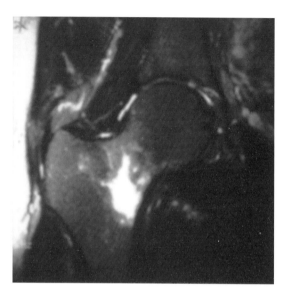

Fig. 8.4
An MRI that shows femoral-neck stress fracture.

The researchers claim that MRI was 100% accurate for diagnosis of stress fracture, compared with bone scan, which had an accuracy of 68% (32% false positives). They recommend that patients who have hip pain undergo radiographs and MRI scans of their hip, and that treatment should be based on the MRI findings.

In the case of a normal radiograph and a positive bone scan (Stage 1), or of sclerosis only (Stage 2), non-weightbearing is required until the hip pain settles. The patient then progresses from partial to full weightbearing on crutches, as his or her symptoms permit. Once he or she is pain free when using crutches, he or she should be allowed to progress to using a walking cane, and then to unprotected weightbearing. A progressive walking, then running, program should be prescribed, and the patient returned to full activity over several months.[6]

The patient who has an undisplaced cortical crack on either the compression or the distraction side of the femoral neck (Stage 3) is treated by way of non-weightbearing on crutches, depending on the pain level, and serial radiographs are taken either every two to three days for the first week or until the rest pain is relieved. He or she then undergoes the same progression as for the Stage 1 and Stage 2 fractures.

For fractures in which there is either any widening or a defect in both cortices (Stage 4), the practitioner undertakes immediate fixation with multiple pins or screws. After radiographic fracture healing and resolution of hip pain by way of unsupported walking, the practitioner may consider removing the fixation. It is recommended that the patient's activity be restricted for at least three months after removal of the hardware in order to enable the bony defects to be filled. During this period, the patient may be allowed to progress to jogging, but should be involved in neither competitive running nor sports. Once clinical and radiographic evidence exists that the postsurgical defects have healed, he or she may resume a gradually increased, progressive, controlled training program in activities such as running, walking, and jumping.[6]

Athletes who present with a displaced femoral neck stress fracture are treated surgically. The practitioner should use closed reduction and internal fixation, whereby either multiple screws or a compression screw with a side plate are used. After the fracture has healed, the practitioner should consider removing the implant, and the patient should undertake a very gradual progression in athletic activity.

In their study, Fullerton and Snowdy[5] had no problems with either prolonged pain or subsequent progression in the patients who were treated nonoperatively. Intermittent discomfort when activity is undertaken can occur for six months up to a year. Avascular necrosis and nonunion are two serious complications that can occur.[11]

Johansson *et al.*[12] followed up twenty-three patients who had a femoral neck stress fracture for an average of 6.5 years after the injury occurred. Sixteen of the patients had been treated by way of internal fixation, and the other seven were treated conservatively. Seven patients

(30%) developed complications for which major surgery was required. The complications were pseudoarthrosis (one patient), avascular necrosis (three patients), and refractures (three patients). Five of the complications occurred in patients who had a displaced fracture, and four of these patients were treated mainly by way of internal fixation. The two other patients had a Type 1 fracture, including periosteal callus without a visible fracture line. One patient was treated by way of internal fixation, and the other had a period of non-weightbearing. The three patients who had avascular necrosis were treated by way of either hip replacement (two patients) or arthrodesis (one patient). Fifty percent of the patients who had a displaced fracture, and 25% who had a Type 1 fracture, decreased their activity level as a consequence of the fracture, mainly because of the pain that activity induced. All the elite athletes in the study decreased their activity to a recreational level after the injury occurred.

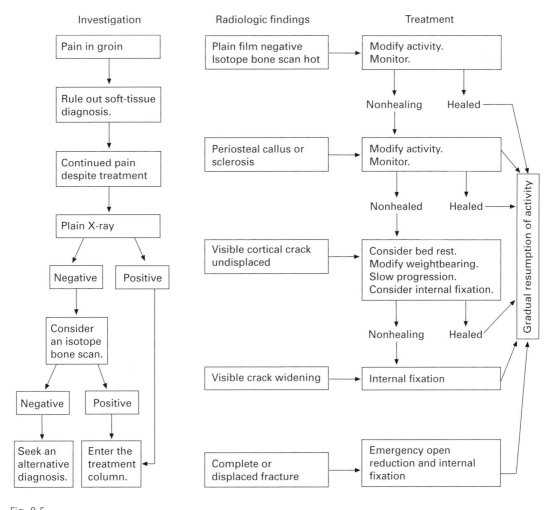

Fig. 8.5

An algorithm for detection and treatment of femoral neck stress fractures (Source: Adapted and reproduced, with permission, from Fullerton LR, Snowdy HA. Femoral neck stress fractures. *American Journal of Sports Medicine* 1988; 16: 365–377).

The researchers conclude that a displaced femoral neck stress fracture is a serious cause of major complications, such as avascular necrosis, refractures, and pseudoarthrosis. They speculate that if there is early diagnosis and treatment, displacement of the fracture may be prevented and the prognosis thereby improved. They emphasize that an isotope bone scan should be conducted when a patient, especially a runner, presents with sudden onset of exertional groin pain and has pain at the extreme of hip movement.

An algorithm for detection and treatment of femoral stress fractures is set out in Fig. 8.5.

The shaft of the femur

Stress fractures of the shaft of the femur have been described among both military recruits and athletes. Volpin *et al.*[13] report a series of 257 consecutive stress fractures among military recruits, and they found that 22.5% of the fractures were femoral. Although relatively speaking the frequency of femoral-shaft stress fractures in athletes is considerably less, there may be a considerable amount of under-diagnosis because of the vague nature of the symptoms.

Also, the stress fractures' location within the femur seems to differ between military recruits and athletes. In their series of thirty-eight femoral stress fractures found among military personnel, Provost and Morris[14] found that more than 50% of the fractures were transverse fractures of the distal third, and that almost half of these were displaced. In the two major studies of femoral stress fractures among athletes,[15,16] eight out of eleven, and six out of seven, femoral shaft stress fractures were located in the proximal femur, specifically either the mid-medial or posteromedial cortex. This finding was consistent with a biomechanical study by Oh and Harris,[17] in which it was shown that a greater strain was applied to the medial–posteromedial cortex of the proximal femur.

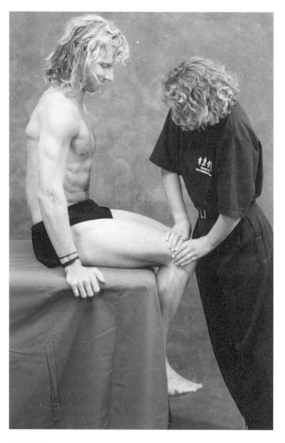

Fig. 8.6
The 'hang test' for femoral stress fractures.

The patient who has a femoral-shaft stress fracture usually presents with vague anterior thigh pain, and very few physical findings. There is often no localized tenderness, and the patient usually has a full range of pain-free movement of the hip and knee joints. The 'hang test', or 'fulcrum test', shown in Fig. 8.6 is believed to be reasonably specific for this type of fracture.[16] In the test, the patient is seated on the edge of a sofa, and has his or her legs dangling over the side. Pressure is then applied over the dorsal aspect of the knee, in a downward direction. The pressure produces markedly increased discomfort in patients who have a stress fracture. The examiner's arm can be placed under the

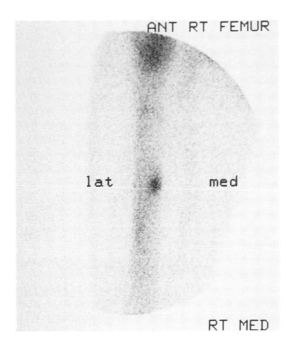

Fig. 8.7
An isotope bone scan of a femoral stress fracture.

distal thigh in order to increase the fulcrum. The test is also used for clinically monitoring the recovery from the stress fracture. When the test is completely negative, it seems to be safe for the patient to gradually return to sport. Johnson *et al.*[16] report that gradual return typically occurs between three and twelve weeks, and that the average is seven weeks. The fracture can be confirmed by way of either an isotope bone scan (Fig. 8.7) or MRI (Fig. 8.8).

At first, treatment of a femoral stress fracture involves having a period of complete rest from activity. A short period of non-weightbearing on crutches may be necessary for pain relief. When the patient is able to walk without pain, and the 'hang test' does not aggravate his or her pain, he or she should be allowed to gradually increase weightbearing activity that consists of slow jogging that is gradually increased in intensity and quantity. The average period from diagnosis to resumption of early jogging is approximately

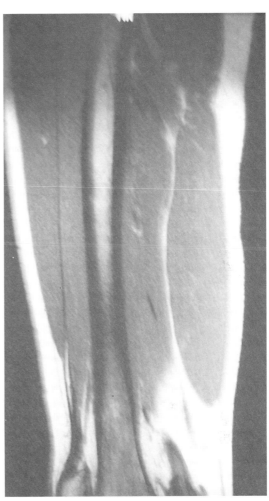

Fig. 8.8
MRI of a femoral stress fracture.

six weeks, and approximately twelve weeks until full resumption of sporting activity.

Reports of displaced femoral stress fractures are occasionally described in the literature.[18] In one case, reported by Dugowson *et al.*,[19] a 32-year-old White female who had had four fibular stress fractures had suffered a fracture that was a displaced femoral shaft, during the thirteenth mile of a half-marathon race. The fracture was successfully fixed internally. The patient's bone-mineral density was well below normal,

SUMMARY

- Stress fracture of the pubic ramus is mainly seen among female distance runners who have a history of amenorrhea and/or an eating disorder.
- Stress fracture of the pubic ramus should be considered for the patient who has exercise-induced groin pain.
- Stress fracture of the femoral neck is a potentially serious condition, because of the possibility of displacement, and of development of avascular necrosis.
- Femoral-neck stress fracture may occur on the superior aspect of the neck, known as the tension or distraction side, or on the inferior aspect of the neck, known as the compression side.
- Stage 1 and Stage 2 fractures are treated by way of close observation and non-weightbearing until the symptoms resolve.
- Stage 3 fractures are treated by way of non-weightbearing and serial radiographs in order to check for displacement.
- Displaced fractures are treated by way of internal fixation.
- The patient who has a stress fracture of the femoral shaft presents with vague anterior thigh pain that is related to exercise.
- The 'hang test' is reasonably specific for this type of fracture.

and she had a history of exercise-associated amenorrhea.

References

1   Noakes TD, Smith JA, Lindenberg G, Willis CE. Pelvic stress fractures in long distance runners. *American Journal of Sports Medicine* 1985; 13: 120–123.

2   Earnst J. Stress fracture of the neck of the femur. *Journal of Trauma* 1964; 4: 71–73.

3   Devas MB. Stress fractures of the femoral neck. *Journal of Bone and Joint Surgery* 1965; 47B: 728–738.

4   Blickenstaff LD, Morris JM. Fatigue fracture of the femoral neck. *Journal of Bone and Joint Surgery* 1966; 48A: 1031–1047.

5   Fullerton LR, Snowdy HA. Femoral neck stress fractures. *American Journal of Sports Medicine* 1988; 16: 365–377.

6   Fullerton LRJ. Femoral neck stress fractures. *Sports Medicine* 1990; 9 (3): 192–197.

7   Milgrom C, Chisin R, Giladi M *et al.* Negative bone scans in impending tibial stress fractures: a report of three cases. *American Journal of Sports Medicine* 1984; 12: 488–491.

8   Sterling JC, Webb RF, Meyers MC, Calvo RD. False negative bone scan in a female runner. *Medicine and Science in Sports and Exercise* 1993; 25 (2): 179–185.

9   Prather JL, Nusynowitz ML, Snowdy HA *et al.* Scintigraphic findings in stress fractures. *Journal of Bone and Joint Surgery* 1977; 59-A: 869–874.

10 Shin AY, Morin WD, Gorman JD, Jones SB, Lapinsky AS. The superiority of magnetic resonance imaging in differentiating the cause of hip pain in endurance athletes. *American Journal of Sports Medicine* 1996; 24 (2): 168–176.

11 Kaltsas D. Stress fractures of the femoral neck in young adults. *Journal of Bone and Joint Surgery* 1981; 63B: 33–37.

12 Johansson C, Ekenman I, Tornkvist H, Eriksson E. Stress fractures of the femoral neck in athletes: the consequence of a delay in diagnosis. *American Journal of Sports Medicine* 1990; 18: 524–528.

13 Volpin G, Hoerer D, Groisman G *et al.* Stress fractures of the femoral neck following strenuous activity. *Journal of Orthopaedics and Traumatology* 1990; 4: 394–398.

14 Provost RA, Morris JM. Fatigue fracture of the femoral shaft. *Journal of Bone and Joint Surgery* 1969; 51-A: 487–498.

15 Hershman EB, Lombardo J, Bergfeld JA. Femoral shaft stress fractures in athletes. *Clinics in Sports Medicine* 1990; 9: 111–119.

16 Johnson AW, Weiss CB, Wheeler DL. Stress fractures of the femoral shaft in athletes – more common than expected: a new clinical test. *American Journal of Sports Medicine* 1994; 22: 248–256.

17 Oh I, Harris WH. Proximal strain distribution in the loaded femur. An *in vitro* comparison of the distributions in the intact femur and after insertion of different hip-replacement femoral components. *Journal of Bone and Joint Surgery* 1978; 60A: 75–85.

18 Clement DB, Ammann W, Taunton JE *et al.* Exercise-induced stress injuries to the femur. *International Journal of Sports Medicine* 1993; 14: 347–352.

19 Dugowson CE, Drinkwater BL, Clark JM. Nontraumatic femur fracture in an oligomentorrheic athlete. *Medicine and Science in Sports and Exercise* 1991; 23: 1323–1325.

Chapter 9

Stress fractures of the lower leg

The most common stress-fracture region is the lower leg, and in most studies the tibia is the most frequent site (see Chapter 1). The fibula is also a common site. The patella and the medial malleolus are relatively uncommon sites. For the practitioner, managing stress fracture of the anterior cortex of the tibia is an interesting challenge.

The patella

Stress fracture of the patella was first described among the athlete population in 1960 by Devas.[1] The researcher described two runners in their twenties who developed pain in the patella region. In the first case, radiographs revealed a vertical fracture of the lateral part of the patella, for which more separation of the fragments was shown three months later. In the second case, there was a transverse fracture of the patella; the fracture was at first undisplaced, but the fragments separated two days later. Both patients were treated operatively, and good results were obtained.

Gerosch *et al.*[2] describes a twenty-year-old recreational athlete who had pain in the region of the patella's inferior pole having had three weeks of intensive soccer practise. During a game, he had suddenly felt a sharp pain while sprinting, which had prevented him from finishing the game. The next day, local swelling had been present, and a tender area was found over the patella's distal third. Active knee extension was painful and weak. Plain radiographs revealed a fracture line in the distal third of the patella, and distraction of the fragments. When an operation was performed, presence of a fracture line was confirmed, and internal fixation was undertaken

using tension-band wiring. Nine months after the surgery, a radiograph revealed bony union, and the internal fixation material was removed.

Teitz and Harrington[3] report two cases of patella stress fracture among adults: one fracture in a sailboarder, the other in a belly dancer. In both cases, the patient's activity required prolonged, isometric quadriceps contraction, whereby the knee was in approximately 30° to 45° of flexion. Mata *et al.*[4] describe a 23-year-old soccer player who had a transverse stress fracture of the patella. Treatment consisted of two weeks' immobilization in a splint, followed by four weeks in a cast, and four weeks' rehabilitation before the patient resumed playing soccer.

Orava *et al.*[5] report five cases of stress fracture of the patella. Four of the fractures occurred transversely in the lower part of the patella, and one fracture occurred longitudinally in the lateral part. Three of the patients were female (an endurance runner, a high jumper and an orienteer), and two were male (a volleyball player and a soccer player). The diagnosis was made two to eight months after the symptoms' onset. Conservative treatment was successful for only one patient; the three other patients were treated surgically, and a good end result was obtained. Drilling of the fracture line was undertaken twice by using tension-band wiring, excision of the lateral fragment was undertaken once, and a bone graft was undertaken once by using K wires and tension band.

A number of reports have been made of patellar stress fracture among adolescent athletes. The fractures are reported among seven boys from eleven to seventeen years of age,[6–9] and in one ten-year-old girl.[8] They include three longitudinal and four transverse stress fractures. The transverse fractures occurred during a basketball match, a soccer match, and high jumping. The longitudinal fractures were caused by running, Japanese fencing, and long-distance walking.

The typical isotope bone scan appearance of a patellar stress fracture is shown in Fig. 9.1.

A patient who has an undisplaced stress fracture should be treated by having a minimum of four weeks' non-weightbearing cast immobilization in knee extension. After the cast has been removed, range-of-motion exercises should be undertaken. The patient may then gradually increase the level of activity over the following three to four weeks. A patient who has a displaced fracture should be treated by way of open reduction and internal fixation.

The tibial plateau

Stress fracture of the tibial plateau is not uncommon in the medial plateau, but is quite rare in the lateral.

Engber[10] reports the cases of thirty-six patients who among them had fifty-seven stress fractures of the medial tibial plateau. The patients complained of pain located on the anteromedial aspect of the tibia's proximal part. When a physical examination was conducted, there was a well-localized area of tenderness to palpation either on the anteromedial aspect of the tibia's proximal end or slightly above the metaphyseal flare. Localized edema in the area of tenderness was present in 75% of the knees. Early plain X-rays were negative unless there had been a delay of more than several weeks between the onset of symptoms and the examination. Treatment consisted of restriction of the patient's activities. Crutches were occasionally used for several days in order to relieve pain. Conservative treatment resulted in all the patients' return to their activity between four and six weeks. In this condition, the main differential diagnosis is pes anserinus bursitis, in which the pain and tenderness occur more posteriorly beneath the fan-like insertions of the sartorius, gracilis, and semitendinosus muscles.

A single case of a stress fracture of the lateral tibial plateau is reported in the literature.[11] A 53-year-old man presented with gradually worsening pain in his right knee. His occupation involved carrying 30 kilograms of glass at a time

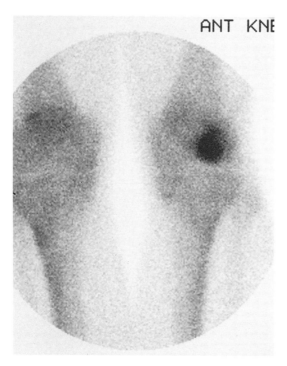

ANT KNE

Fig. 9.1
The isotope bone scan appearance of a patellar stress fracture.

under his right arm, for installation in buildings. There was tenderness over the lateral tibial condyle, but no swelling. The patient was noted as having valgus angulation of 8° in the affected leg, and of 1° in his left knee. A plain radiograph revealed a radiolucent line that extended 1.5 centimeters longitudinally from the lateral plateau. The patient's pain failed to settle after five weeks of crutch ambulation, and arthroscopy was undertaken. The articular surface of the lateral tibial plateau showed widespread fibrillation, and a crack that ran to and fro on the posterior third. The fracture was fixed internally by using a cancellous screw. No cast brace was applied after surgery, and weightbearing was allowed as tolerated. Three months after the surgery, the patient was asymptomatic, and a radiograph revealed that the fracture had healed.

The tibial shaft

The tibia is the most common stress-fracture site. Although distinguishing stress fracture from other common causes of exercise-related shin pain may present a diagnostic challenge, management of most tibial stress fractures is relatively straightforward. There is, however, a subgroup of tibial stress fractures, ones that affect the anterior cortex of the tibia's middle third, which are especially prone to nonunion, and will be considered separately.

Shin pain is an extremely common complaint among athletes. In the past, the term 'shin splints' was used for describing the pain along the shin's medial border that was commonly experienced by runners. However, it is important there be a more precise pathologic diagnosis, so the term 'shin splints' should be avoided.

Shin pain usually occurs in one or more of the following three anatomic structures.[12]

1. Bone: A continuum of bone damage exists, from bone strain to stress reaction and stress fracture.

2. Tenoperiosteum: Inflammation develops at the aponeurotic insertion of muscle, particularly the tibialis posterior and soleus, and fascia to the medial border of the tibia.

3. Muscle compartments: These involve the anterior compartment syndrome and deep posterior compartment syndrome.

These three abnormalities can usually be distinguished on the basis of history, examination, and investigations. It is important it be remembered that two or three of these conditions may coexist. It is not uncommon, for example, that a stress fracture develops in a patient who has chronic tenoperiostitis. Tenoperiostitis and muscle compartment syndrome often occur together. This overlap of conditions may be related to a common biomechanic abnormality, such as excessive pronation. Guidelines for differentiating between the three main sites of shin pain are set out in Table 9.1.

The most important aspect of any clinical assessment is the history. In the case of the athlete who has shin pain, the history's most important aspect is the relationship of pain to exercise. If the pain improves after the athlete has warmed up and undertaken continued exercise, it is most likely the problems are tenoperiosteal. If the pain worsens when exercise is undertaken and a feeling of tightness accompanies it, compartment syndrome may be present. Pain that comes on after a certain length of time and that gradually increases is likely to be bony in origin.

The athlete who has a stress fracture of the tibia presents with gradual onset of shin pain that is aggravated by exercise. The pain may occur when the patient is walking or at rest, or even at night. Examination reveals localized tenderness over the tibia, typically on the posteromedial border of the lower third, which is the most common site. There may be some swelling or thickening as a result of callus at the site. Biomechanic examination may reveal either a rigid cavus foot that is incapable of absorbing

Table 9.1 Guidelines for differentiating between the three main sites of shin pain

Site	Pain	Related to exercise	Associated features	Tenderness	Investigations
Bone	Localized Acute or sharp	Constant or increasing Worse with impact	Night ache May be increased in the morning	Bony	X-ray Isotope bone scan
Tenoperiosteum	Medial border of tibia Variable intensity	Decreases as warms up	Worse in the morning and after exercise	Medial tibular border at site of muscle attachment	Isotope bone scan
Muscle compartment	Ache Tightness Claudicant type	Increases with exercise Decreases with rest	Occasionally muscle weakness or sensory symptoms	Usually minimal	Compartment pressure testing Isotope bone scan

Source: Adapted and reproduced, with permission, from Brukner P, Khan K. Clinical Sports Medicine. *Sydney: McGraw-Hill, 1993: 405 (table 24.1).*

load or an excessively pronating foot whereby muscle fatigue is caused. For athletes who have excessively pronated feet, the muscles of the superficial and deep compartments are required to contract harder and longer eccentrically in order to resist pronation after heel strike. On toe-off, the muscles then work hard concentrically in order to accelerate supination. When the athlete is fatigued, these muscles fail to provide the normal degree of shock absorption and may thereby contribute to development of bone stress, and ultimately to occurrence of a stress fracture. Tightening of calf muscles, which commonly occurs as a result of hard training, will restrict ankle dorsiflexion and increase the tendency for excessive pronation, thereby leading to increased internal rotation of the tibia.

In many cases, a clinical diagnosis of tibial stress fracture can be made on the basis of a history of exercise-related bone pain that is localized to the lower third of the tibia and is associated with a focal area of tenderness at the posteromedial border of the tibia. If more confirmation of the clinical diagnosis is required, investigations can be conducted. Although plain radiography may be undertaken, Matheson *et al.*[13] report that on plain films, only 10% of their subjects showed evidence of stress fracture. Plain X-rays may reveal a faint crack in the tibia or, more commonly, evidence of periosteal new-bone formation (Fig. 9.2). Conducting an isotope bone scan may help confirm presence of a stress fracture. On an isotope bone scan, the typical appearance of a tibial stress fracture (Fig. 9.3) is of a focal fusiform area of increased uptake that corresponds to the site of the symptoms and the tenderness. This area may be either isolated, as in Fig. 9.3, or superimposed on a typical bone-scan appearance of tenoperiostitis. Compartment syndrome also has a characteristic appearance on an isotope bone scan of the deep posterior compartment (Fig. 9.4) and the anterior

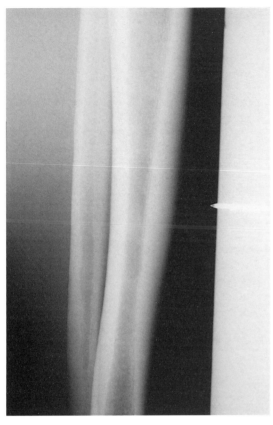

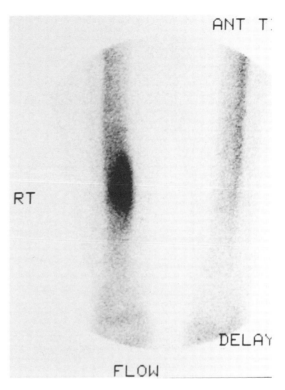

Fig. 9.3
The typical appearance of an isotope bone scan of a tibial stress fracture.

Fig. 9.2
A plain radiograph of a tibial stress fracture that shows periosteal reaction.

compartment (Fig. 9.5). The typical MRI appearance of stress fracture is shown in Fig. 9.6.

A combination of clinical features and a focal area of increased uptake on bone scan are sufficient in most cases for the clinician to make a diagnosis of tibial stress fracture. However, without actually visualizing the fracture, the clinician can never be totally confident that he or she is dealing with a stress fracture as opposed to a stress reaction. In most cases, this question is not of clinical significance, because treatment is the same and the patient's healing is monitored clinically by way of assessment of pain and local tenderness. In the case of an elite athlete who

has a deadline of upcoming competition, a CT scan can be conducted in order to differentiate between stress reaction and stress fracture. In this situation, lack of evidence on CT would indicate that a stress reaction rather than a stress fracture is present, and the clinician would thereby be enabled to predict that the athlete will return to sport much earlier than he or she would were a stress fracture present. The clinician can also be more aggressive in prescribing a rehabilitation program of modified activity. A typical CT appearance of a tibial stress fracture is shown in Fig. 9.7.

Treatment of tibial stress fracture involves at first a period of rest (in which a period of non-weightbearing on crutches for pain relief is sometimes required) before the pain settles. The

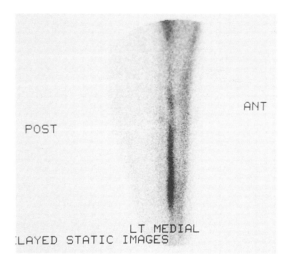

Fig. 9.4
The typical bone-scan appearance of deep posterior compartment syndrome.

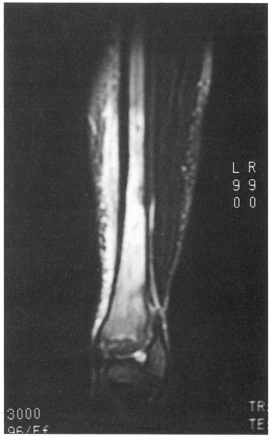

Fig. 9.6
The MRI appearance of a tibial stress fracture.

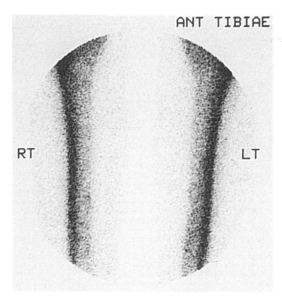

Fig. 9.5
The typical bone-scan appearance of anterior compartment syndrome.

patient should continue to rest from the aggravating activity until the bony tenderness disappears, and this usually occurs between four and eight weeks. Alternative activity as described in Chapter 5 should be undertaken. The aggravating activity should be gradually resumed along the lines described previously, in Chapter 5. Although the time to return to full activity varies considerably between fractures, and probably depends on the stage of each fracture in the continuum of bone stress, the average period is eight to twelve weeks.

Once the patient is pain free when walking and has no bony tenderness, over the following

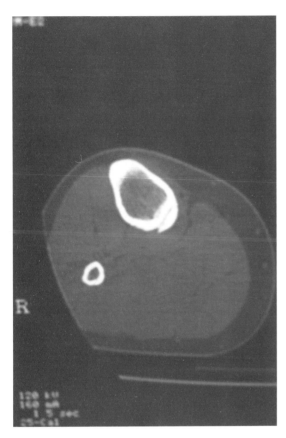

Fig. 9.7
The CT-scan appearance of a tibial stress fracture.

It is important that the factors that have precipitated the stress fracture be determined. These factors are discussed in Chapter 3.

Use of a pneumatic brace (an Aircast) has been described in three studies.[14–16] In these studies, a markedly reduced return-to-activity time has been shown, compared with an average time in two of the three studies,[14,15] and compared with a 'traditional treatment' group in the third study.[16] In the lastmentioned study, the brace group returned to full, unrestricted activity in an average of twenty-one days, compared with seventy-seven days for the traditional group. Once a stress fracture has clinically healed, the athlete is advised to use the brace during both practise and competition.

It is believed that the brace unloads the tibia by compressing the lower leg, redistributing the forces, and decreasing the amount of tibial bowing.[15]

Swenson and colleagues[16] propose that the pneumatic leg brace shifts a portion of the weightbearing load from the tibia to the soft tissue, which results in less impact loading when the athlete is walking, hopping, and running. They believe that stabilization of the stress fracture contributes to earlier pain-free walking, and to an earlier completion of a functional progression program.

An unusual tibial stress fracture has been reported. Clayer *et al.*[17] present two cases in which the fracture ran longitudinally in the distal one-third of the tibia. In one case, a 24-year-old man developed pain while playing golf, and in the second case, a 55-year-old woman developed pain while undertaking home duties. In both the cases, although plain radiographs were normal, isotope bone scans showed increased uptake in the lower tibia. CT scans demonstrated a longitudinal fracture, including callus formation. Both the patients healed clinically after having restriction of activities. In previous reports of this type of fracture,[18–21] all the patients were older (forty-five to sixty-one years old). This type of fracture has subsequently been

month there should be a gradual progression of the quantity and quality of the exercise undertaken. During the enforced layoff period, alternative exercises such as swimming, cycling, and water running should be undertaken in order to maintain aerobic fitness. During the rehabilitation period, the patient may complain of pain in the affected area, and this is frequently the result of soft-tissue thickening that is often found distal to the fracture site. We have had success treating this soft-tissue thickening by using deep-massage therapy. For these fractures, the general principles of return to activity after a stress fracture has occurred should be followed.

reported by Krauss and Van Meter,[22] Keating *et al.*,[23] Jeske *et al.*,[24] Umans and Kaye,[25] and Feydy *et al.*[26]

In their report of six cases, Umans and Kaye[25] describe this fracture's MRI appearances. In each case, MRI revealed linear marrow signal abnormalities that were oriented along the long axis of the tibial shaft. Endosteal callus and periosteal callus were identified on axial images. In all cases, MRI clearly showed a fracture line that extended through one cortex, with abnormal signal in both the marrow cavity and the adjacent soft tissues, which indicated edema.

Feydy *et al.*[26] compare the performance of CT and MRI in diagnosing longitudinal stress fractures of the tibia among fifteen patients. The CT and MRI techniques enabled the fracture line to be detected in 82% and 73% of the cases, respectively. However, the MRI technique had a sensitivity that was markedly higher than that of CT in detection of bone-marrow edema (73% versus 18%) and of soft-tissue lesions (87% versus 9%).

The anterior cortex of the tibia

Fractures of the anterior cortex of mid shaft of the tibia have to be considered separately, because they are prone to delayed union, nonunion, and complete fracture. These fractures were first described in 1956 by Burrows,[27] among ballet dancers. In Burrows' series, four of the five dancers returned to activity on an average of fifteen months after diagnosis, and the fifth dancer sustained a comminuted fracture of the mid-tibia two weeks after the onset of symptoms. That fracture healed after fourteen months, after the dancer spent eight months in a long-leg cast. Friedenberg[28] and Stanitski *et al.*[29] also report cases of nonunion of stress fracture of the anterior tibial cortex. Brahms *et al.*[30] present a case report in which a spontaneous

complete fracture through the stress fracture area occurred.

Green *et al.*[31] present six cases of stress fracture of the anterior cortex of the middle third of the tibia that failed to unite by way of conservative management. The patients' average age was 16.7 years, and five of the six stress fractures became a complete fracture. The five patients who sustained a complete fracture were immobilized for an average of 6.6 months. One patient was treated by using electromagnetic stimulation. Three of the patients underwent excision of the nonunion, including addition of iliac bone grafts on an average of eleven months after the stress fracture was first diagnosed. One patient underwent simple biopsy of the lesion, and the fifth patient underwent open reduction and internal fixation of his second complete fracture. The researchers postulate that the reason for the high incidence of nonunion in their series and in their previous reports was that the mid-shaft of the tibia is loaded under tension rather than under compression, and that it was probable that the fractures were the result of tensile forces more than of compression forces. They recommend that whether complete or not, the fractures be treated by way of immobilization, and that if there is no radiographic evidence of healing after four to six months the practitioner seriously consider internal fixation and bone grafting.

Blank[32] reports five cases of tibial transverse stress fractures, three of which were in the anterior middle third of the tibia. One patient developed a complete fracture line through the stress injury. Interestingly, in three of the cases, isotope bone scans revealed no evidence of increased uptake at the fracture site. Blank postulates that the lack of evidence of radionuclide uptake indicated nonunion.

Rettig *et al.*[33] present eight cases of competitive basketballers who had a stress fracture of the anterolateral cortex of the tibia's mid shaft. All eight patients were treated by having rest and/or therapy that involved a pulsed electromagnetic field. Although one of the patients required a bone-grafting procedure, all eight of the patients showed complete healing and were able to return to full activity after an average of 8.7 months of treatment. Overall, the average time from first symptoms to return to competition was 12.5 months. The researchers suggest that because the anterior tibial cortex is located subcutaneously, its hypovascularity may be a factor that predisposes athletes to delayed union.

Orava *et al.*[34] report seventeen cases of this stress fracture, in which the mean age was twenty-six. Six of the athletes were at international level, the others national. All seventeen athletes were at first treated by having rest from physical activity, and eight of them showed clinical healing in three to ten months (an average of six months). Nine of the athletes progressed to either delayed union or nonunion whereby operative treatment was required. The surgery involved transverse drilling of the hypertrophied anterior cortex in order to enhance bone formation. In the surgically treated cases, the postoperative recovery time was on average six months.

A patient who has a stress fracture of the anterior cortex of the medial third of the tibia presents with diffuse, dull pain that is aggravated by physical activity. The bone is tender to palpation at the fracture site, and periosteal thickening as evidenced by a palpable lump may be present if the symptoms have been present for some months.

In the phase of acute stress fracture, plain radiographs are often normal, although periosteal thickening and callus will eventually be seen in most cases. Isotope bone scan (Fig. 9.8) reveals a discrete focal area of increased activity in the anterior cortex.

These stress fractures almost inevitably progress to nonunion, and the patient does not usually present to the practitioner until this

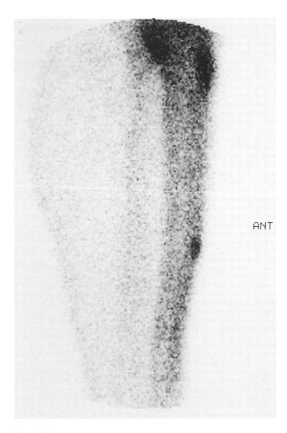

ANT

Fig. 9.8
The bone-scan appearance of a stress fracture of the anterior cortex of the tibia.

stage, at which the radiographic appearance is of a defect in the anterior cortex that is termed the 'dreaded black line' (Fig. 9.9). This appearance is due to bony resorption, and indicates nonunion. At this stage, the isotope bone scan will often fail to show any increase in uptake, and the patient will frequently have only minimal symptoms and may be fully participating in sport.

Biopsies have shown presence of dense cortical bone and empty lacunae that lack osteophytes, with sparse granulation tissue at the nonunion site.[27-29] Some researchers describe

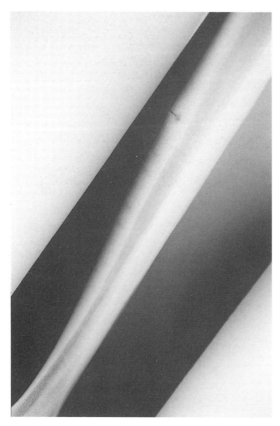

Fig. 9.9
A plain radiograph of nonunion of a stress fracture of the anterior cortex of the tibia (the 'dreaded black line').

the histologic appearance as being typical of a pseudoarthrosis.[34,35]

It is believed that the mid-anterior cortex of the tibia is vulnerable to nonunion for two reasons: that the area has a relatively poor blood supply, and that it is an area that is under tension because of morphologic bowing of the tibia. Excessive anterior-tibial bowing is often noted in association with this type of fracture.

In the literature, anecdotal reports indicate that only a relatively small proportion of these fractures will heal clinically and radiographically by way of conservative management that consists of an extended period of cast immobilization. Other forms of treatment that

various researchers advocate include pulsed electromagnetic stimulation,[33] surgical excision and bone grafting,[22,31] and transverse drilling at the fracture site.[34]

Chang and Harris[36] describe five cases in which the patients were treated by way of intramedullary tibial nailing. Two excellent and three good results were obtained.

Pulsed electromagnetic fields,[37–44] direct electric currents,[45–48] and capacitively coupled electric fields[45,46,49–52] have all been shown to have a positive effect on healing of nonunion of traumatic fractures. Although no proper study has been undertaken in order to evaluate the efficacy of any of these treatments in management of nonunion of stress fractures, it is reasonable to assume that the treatments may be of some benefit.

For both the acute stress fracture and the established nonunion as denoted by presence of a 'dreaded black line' on plain radiograph, our recommended management is avoidance of the aggravating activity, use of a long pneumatic leg brace, and electrical stimulation for ten hours per day. Monitoring of the fracture's healing should be both clinical and radiographic. Athletes should be advised not to return to activity until evidence exists of cortical bridging on radiography. If after four to six months there is no evidence of healing either clinically or radiologically, the practitioner should undertake drilling at the fracture site, insertion of an intramedullary rod, or bone grafting.

Recently, we surgically treated five patients who had this condition by 'scalloping out' the area of bony cortex that involved the fracture. All the patients did well, and on average returned to full activity two months after surgery.

The fibula

Fibular stress fractures are not seen as frequently as tibial stress fractures. Because the fibula has a minimal role in weightbearing, it is believed that fibular stress fracture develops as a result of muscle traction and torsional forces placed through the bone. For the athlete who has excessive subtalar pronation, the peroneal muscles are forced to contract harder and longer during toe-off.

Patients will complain of lateral leg or ankle pain, and occasionally of swelling. Examination may reveal local tenderness and pain when the fibula is sprung proximal to the stress-fracture site. Differential diagnosis of fibular stress fractures includes peroneal compartment syndrome. An isotope bone scan can be conducted in order to confirm the diagnosis.

This type of stress fracture is usually not as painful when weightbearing is undertaken compared with tibial stress fracture. The patient is treated symptomatically by way of rest from activity until the bony tenderness settles. He or she should then have a gradual increase in the amount of activity. Soft-tissue tightness should be corrected. This injury is often associated with a biomechanical abnormality, such as excessive pronation or excessive supination.

Although most stress fractures are in the distal third of the fibula, proximal stress fractures have also been described.[53–56] In the literature, two other unusual fibular stress fractures are reported: a stress fracture that was associated with distal tibiofibular synostosis,[57] and delayed union of a fibular stress fracture secondary to rotational malunion of a lateral malleolar fracture.[58]

The medial malleolus

Stress fractures of the medial malleolus were first described by Shelbourne *et al.*[59] The researchers formulated the following criteria for diagnosing this type of stress fracture. The patient presents with tenderness over the medial malleolus, as well as ankle effusion, having for several weeks experienced discomfort and pain during running and jumping activities before

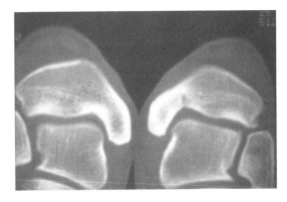

Fig. 9.10
A plain radiograph of stress fracture of the medial malleolus.

experiencing an acute episode that results in their seeking medical attention. Although the fracture line is frequently vertical from the junction of the tibial plafond and the medial malleolus (Fig. 9.10), it may arch obliquely from the junction to the distal tibial metaphysis. If there are clinical signs and a clinical history, and if the fracture line is not detected on radiographs, a bone scan should be conducted. If on the bone scan there is increased uptake in the area of the medial malleolus, the injury fits the criteria for a stress fracture of the medial malleolus.

In their paper, Shelbourne *et al.*[59] present six case histories of patients who had a medial-malleolar stress fracture. Three of the patients had a fracture line that could be seen on a plain radiograph, and they were treated by way of open reduction and internal fixation. Although the other three patients had a normal radiograph, their bone scan revealed increased uptake over the medial malleolus. These three patients were treated by way of immobilization in either a cast or a pneumatic leg brace.

Shelbourne and colleagues postulate that when the forefoot is pronated, the navicular bone moves into an abducted position relative to the talar head. This imposes an internal rotational force on the talus that is subsequently transmitted to the medial malleolus. The rotation of the medial malleolus then causes tibial rotation. There is therefore a direct relationship between forefoot pronation and internal tibial rotation. This relationship is also noted when an athlete attempts to rotate the tibia externally while the forefoot is planted in pronation. External tibial rotation is then prevented by the talus, whereby an opposing rotational force is distributed on to the medial malleolus. As a result of repetitive, overloading cyclic stress, a microfracture may develop at the junction of the medial malleolus and the tibial plafond.

In Shelbourne's cases, his surgically treated patients began to undertake motion shortly after fixation, progressed to running activities within six weeks, and fully participated in their sport after eight weeks. The nonsurgically treated patients were allowed to have unlimited ambulation in a pneumatic leg brace, and also progressed to full participation after six to eight weeks.

Rieder *et al.*[60] report a case of nonunion of a medial malleolar stress fracture. In this paper, the researchers note that for acute fractures of the medial malleolus that were treated conservatively, the nonunion rate was as high as 10% to 15% as a result of inadequate closed reduction and interposition of periosteum. In this case, for more than two years the patient had pain in the area that had not been diagnosed correctly as being a stress fracture.

Schils *et al.*[61] describe seven patients who had a medial malleolar stress fracture, and in their study especially paid attention to the imaging features. The early radiographic findings included one or two linear areas of hyperlucency that were between 2 and 15 millimeters long. In five of the patients, the areas originated at the medial malleolus – tibial plafond junction,

and were vertically oriented; in one patient, the fissure arched obliquely through the medial malleolus; and one patient had a normal radiograph. The fissure was best seen on the anteroposterior radiograph. In three of the patients, well-circumscribed lytic lesions surrounded the fissure. In two of the seven patients, a complete vertical fracture of the medial malleolus occurred that extended from the tibial plafond to the medial cortex. For the two patients in whom the medial malleolus was completely fractured, one was treated in a cast for eight weeks and returned to full athletic activities five months later, and the other sustained a fracture while jogging seven months after the open reduction and internal fixation of the medial malleolus. Open reduction and internal fixation were again undertaken, and clinical and radiographic evidence and healing were seen eight months later. Two of the other five patients were treated by way of open reduction and internal fixation of the medial malleolus, and the other three were placed in either a cast or a pneumatic leg brace for six weeks.

Orava *et al.*[62] report a series of eight patients who had a medial malleolar stress fracture. The early radiographs revealed that the fracture was present in only three of the patients. For the other five patients, the diagnosis was made by way of an isotope bone scan, and was confirmed by way of a CT scan, MRI, or a subsequent plain radiograph. One vertical fracture was at first treated by way of compression using AO screws. Two of the patients had delayed healing and symptoms for eight and twelve months. These fracture sites were drilled, and the fractures healed four and five months after drilling. All the five patients who were managed nonoperatively healed within five months (an average of four months).

We recommend that an undisplaced or a minimally displaced stress fracture of the medial malleolus be treated conservatively in a

SUMMARY

- A stress fracture of the patella may be either a transverse or a longitudinal undisplaced fracture and should be treated by way of cast immobilization.
- The tibia is the most common stress-fracture site among athletes.
- Bony pain can be differentiated from the other causes of shin pain on the basis of the pain's relationship to exercise.
- Most tibial stress fractures will heal if the patient has four to eight weeks' rest from the aggravating activity.
- Stress fractures of the anterior cortex of the tibia are prone to nonunion and should be treated by way of either immobilization or internal fixation.
- Fibular stress fractures are reasonably common, and most of them heal uneventfully.
- Stress fractures of the medial malleolus are rare. Undisplaced fractures should be treated in a pneumatic leg brace (Aircast); displaced fractures require reduction and internal fixation.

pneumatic leg brace for six weeks. A displaced fracture or a fracture that progresses to nonunion should be treated operatively.

References

1 Devas MB. Stress fractures of the patella. *Journal of Bone and Joint Surgery* 1960; 42-B: 71–74.

2 Gerosch JG, Castro WHM, Jantier C. Stress fracture of the patella. *American Journal of Sports Medicine* 1989; 17 (4): 579–580.

3 Teitz CC, Harrington RM. Patellar stress fracture. *American Journal of Sports Medicine* 1992; 20: 761–765.

4 Mata SG, Grande MM, Ovejero AH. Transverse stress fracture of the patella. *Clinical Journal of Sport Medicine* 1996; 6: 259–261.

5 Orava S, Taimela S, Kvist M *et al.* Diagnosis and treatment of stress fracture of the patella in athletes. *Knee Surgery Sports Traumatology Arthroscopy* 1996; 4 (4): 206–211.

6 Hanel DP, Burdge RE. Consecutive indirect patella fractures in an adolescent basketball player. *American Journal of Sports Medicine* 1981; 9: 327–329.

7 Dickason JM, Fox JM. Fracture of the patella due to overuse syndrome in a child: a case report. *American Journal of Sports Medicine* 1982; 10: 248–249.

8 Iwaya T, Takatori I. Lateral longitudinal stress fractures of the patella: report of three cases. *Journal of Pediatric Orthopedics* 1985; 5: 73–75.

9 Pietu G, Hauet P. Stress fracture of the patella: a case report. *Acta Orthopedica Scandinavica* 1995; 66 (5): 481–482.

10 Engber WD. Stress fractures of the medial tibial plateau. *Journal of Bone and Joint Surgery* 1977; 59-A: 767–769.

11 Mizuta H, Takagi K, Sakata H. An unusual stress fracture of the lateral tibial plateau. *Archives of Orthopaedics and Trauma Surgery* 1993; 112: 96–98.

12 Brukner P, Khan K. *Clinical Sports Medicine*. Sydney: McGraw-Hill, 1993.

13 Matheson GO, Clement DB, McKenzie DC *et al.* Stress fractures in athletes: a study of 320 cases. *American Journal of Sports Medicine* 1987; 15: 46–58.

14 Dickson TB, Kichline PD. Functional management of stress fractures in female athletes using a pneumatic leg brace. *American Journal of Sports Medicine* 1987; 15: 86–89.

15 Whitelaw GP, Wetzler MJ, Levy AS, Segal D, Bissonett K. A pneumatic leg brace for the treatment of tibial stress fractures. *Clinical Orthopedic Related Research* 1991; 270: 302–305.

16 Swenson EJ, DeHaven KE, Sebastienelli WJ *et al.* The effect of a pneumatic leg brace on return to play in athletes with tibial stress fractures. *American Journal of Sports Medicine* 1997; 25 (3): 322–328.

17 Clayer M, Krishnan J, Lee WK, Tamblyn P. Longitudinal stress fracture of the tibia: two cases. *Clinical Radiology* 1992; 46: 401–404.

18 Allen GJ. Longitudinal stress fractures of the tibia: diagnosis with CT. *Radiology* 1988; 167: 799–801.

19 Miniaci A, McLaren AC, Haddad RG. Longitudinal stress fracture of the tibia: case report. *Journal of the Canadian Association of Radiologists* 1988; 39: 221–223.

20 Goupille P, Giraudet-LeQuintrec JS, Hilliquin P, Job-Deslander C, Menkes CJ. Fracture de contrainte

longitudinale du tibia: a propos d'une observation. *Revue de Rhumatisme* 1989; 56: 705–708.

21 Mazzonetto M, De Antoni M, Vendeniati E. Frattura longitudinale della tibia da stress: diagnosi con TC. *Radiology Medica* 1989; 77: 411–412.

22 Krauss MD, Van Meter CD. A longitudinal tibial stress fracture. *Orthopedic Reviews* 1994; 23 (2): 163–166.

23 Keating JF, Beggs I, Thorpe GW. Three cases of longitudinal stress fracture of the tibia. *Acta Orthopedica Scandinavica* 1995; 66 (1): 41–42.

24 Jeske JM, Lomasney LM, Demos TC, Vade A, Bielski RJ. Longitudinal tibial stress fracture. *Orthopedics* 1996; 19 (3): 263.

25 Umans HR, Kaye JJ. Longitudinal stress fractures of the tibia: diagnosis by magnetic resonance imaging. *Skeletal Radiology* 1996; 25 (4): 319–324.

26 Feydy A, Draper JL, Beret E *et al.* Longitudinal stress fractures of the tibia – comparative study of CT and MR imaging. *European Radiology* 1998; 8 (4): 598–602.

27 Burrows HJ. Fatigue infraction of the middle of the tibia in ballet dancers. *Journal of Bone and Joint Surgery* 1956; 38-B: 83–94.

28 Friedenberg ZB. Fatigue fractures of the tibia. *Clinical Orthopaedics* 1971; 76: 111–115.

29 Stanitski CL, McMaster JH, Scranton PE. On the nature of stress fractures. *American Journal of Sports Medicine* 1978; 6: 391–396.

30 Brahms MA, Fumich RM, Ippolita VD. Atypical stress fracture of tibia in a professional athlete. *American Journal of Sports Medicine* 1980; 8: 131–132.

31 Green NE, Rogers RA, Lipscomb B. Nonunions of stress fractures of the tibia. *American Journal of Sports Medicine* 1985; 13: 171–176.

32 Blank S. Transverse tibial stress fractures: a special problem. *American Journal of Sports Medicine* 1987; 15: 597–607.

33 Rettig AC, Shelbourne KD, McCarroll JR, Bisesi M, Watts J. The natural history and treatment of delayed union and non-union stress fractures of the anterior cortex of the tibia. *American Journal of Sports Medicine* 1988; 16: 250–255.

34 Orava S, Karpakka J, Hulkko A *et al.* Diagnosis and treatment of stress fractures located at the mid-tibial shaft in athletes. *International Journal of Sports Medicine* 1991; 12: 419–422.

35 Rolf C, Ekenman I, Tornqvist H, Gad A. The anterior stress fracture of the tibia: an atrophic pseudoarthrosis. *Scandinavian Journal of Medicine and Science in Sports* 1997; 7 (4): 249–252.

36 Chang PS, Harris RM. Intramedullary nailing for chronic tibial stress fractures: a review of five cases. *American Journal of Sports Medicine* 1996; 24 (5): 688–692.

37 Bassett CAL, Pawluk RJ, Becker RO. Augmentation of bone repair by inductively coupled electromagnetic fields. *Science* 1974; 184: 575–577.

38 Bassett CAL, Mitchell SN, Norton L, Pilla A. A non-operative salvage of surgically-resistant pseudarthroses and non-unions by pulsating electromagnetic fields: a preliminary report. *Clinical Orthopaedics* 1977; 124: 128.

39 Bassett CAL, Mitchell SN, Norton L. Repair of non-union by pulsing electromagnetic fields. *Acta Orthopedica Belge* 1978; 44: 706–724.

40 Bassett CAL, Mitchell SN, Gaston SR. Treatment of ununited tibial diaphyseal fractures with pulsing electromagnetic fields. *Journal of Bone and Joint Surgery* 1981; 63-A: 511–523.

41 Barker AT, Dixon RA, Sharrard WJ, Sutcliffe ML. Pulsed magnetic field therapy for tibial non-union: interim results of a double-blind trial. *Lancet* 1984; 1: 994–996.

42 O'Connor BT. Pulsed magnetic field therapy for tibial non-union. *Lancet* 1984; 2: 171–172.

43 De Haas WG, Beaupre A, Cameron H, English E. The Canadian experience with pulsed magnetic fields in the treatment of ununited tibial stress fractures. *Clinical Orthopedics* 1986; 208: 55–58.

44 Sharrard WJW. A double-blind trial of pulsed electromagnetic fields for delayed union of tibial fractures. *Journal of Bone and Joint Surgery* 1990; 72-B (3): 347–355.

45 Brighton CT, Black J, Friedenberg ZB *et al.* A multicenter study of the treatment of non-union with constant direct current. *Journal of Bone and Joint Surgery* 1981; 63-A: 2–13.

46 Brighton CT, Shaman P, Heppenstall RB *et al.* Tibial nonunion treated with direct current, capacitive coupling, or bone graft. *Clinical Orthopaedics* 1995; 321: 223–234.

47 Esterhai JL, Brighton CT, Heppenstall RB, Alavi A, Desai AG. Detection of synovial pseudarthrosis by 99mTc scintigraphy: application to treatment of traumatic non-union with constant direct current. *Clinical Orthopaedics* 1981; 161: 15–23.

48 Parnell EJ, Simons RB. The effect of electrical stimulation in the treatment of non-union of the tibia. *Journal of Bone and Joint Surgery* 1991; 73-B: S178.

49 Brighton CT, Pollock SR. Treatment of non-union of the tibia with a capacitively coupled electric field. *Journal of Traumatology* 1984; 24: 153.

50 Brighton CT, Pollock SR. Treatment of recalcitrant nonunion with a capacitively coupled electric field: a preliminary report. *Journal of Bone and Joint Surgery* 1985; 67-A: 577–585.

51 Brighton CT, McCluskey WP. The early response of bone cells in culture to a capacitively coupled electric field. *Trans Biolectric Repair and Growth Society* 1983; 3: 10.

52 Scott G, King JB. A prospective, double blind trial of electrical capacitive coupling in the treatment of non-union of long bones. *Journal of Bone and Joint Surgery* 1994; 76-A (6): 820–826.

53 Blair WF, Hanley SR. Stress fracture of the proximal fibula. *American Journal of Sports Medicine* 1980; 8: 212–213.

54 Oliveri M, Lazzoni P, Pratho N, Gambaro GA. A case of bilateral fibular stress fracture in a jogger. *Italian Journal of Sports Traumatology* 1989; 11 (3): 227–231.

55 Strudwick WJ, Goodman SB. Proximal fibular stress fracture in an aerobic dancer: a case report. *American Journal of Sports Medicine* 1992; 20 (4): 481–482.

56 Lacroix H, Keeman JN. An unusual stress fracture of the fibula in a long-distance runner. *Archives of Orthopaedics and Trauma Surgery* 1992; 111 (5): 289–290.

57 Kottmeier SA, Hanks GA, Kalenak A. Fibular stress fracture associated with distal tibiofibular synostosis in an athlete: a case report and literature review. *Clinical Orthopaedics* 1992; 281: 195–198.

58 Guille JT, Lipton GE, Bowen JR, Uthaman U. Delayed union following stress fracture of the distal fibula secondary to rotational malunion of lateral malleolar fracture. *American Journal of Orthopedics* 1997; 26 (6): 442–445.

59 Shelbourne KD, Fisher DA, Rettig AC, McCarroll JR. Stress fractures of the medial malleolus. *American Journal of Sports Medicine* 1988; 16: 60–63.

60 Rieder B, Falconier R, Yurkofsky J. Nonunion of a medial malleolus stress fracture: a case report. *American Journal of Sports Medicine* 1993; 21 (3): 478–481.

61 Schils JP, Andrish JT, Piraino DW *et al*. Medial malleolar stress fractures in seven patients: review of the clinical and imaging features. *Radiology* 1992; 185 (1): 219–221.

62 Orava S, Karpakka J, Taimela S *et al*. Stress fracture of the medial malleolus. *Journal of Bone and Joint Surgery (Am)* 1995; 77 (3): 362–365.

Chapter 10

Stress fractures of the foot and ankle

The first types of stress fracture that were described in the literature were metatarsal stress fractures, and because they were first described among the military, they were termed 'march fracture'. They are also common among runners and dancers. Although most stress fractures of the foot are relatively straightforward, several require either a prolonged period of immobilization or special treatment because of their propensity for either delayed union or nonunion.

The talus

Two types of stress fracture of the talus are reported. The first type, talar neck stress fracture, is mainly reported among military recruits, and one of the fractures was associated with tarsal coalition.[1] Only one case of talar neck stress fracture is described in an athlete.[2] The second type of talar stress fracture is a vertical lateral body fracture near the junction of the body with the lateral process of the talus.[3–5]

Campbell and Warnekros[2] report the case of a 58-year-old, male long-distance runner who presented with a painful swollen ankle. Examination revealed an area of pain and swelling near the anterior talofibular and calcaneofibular ligaments. When both dorsiflexion and plantar flexion were undertaken, pain radiated to the posterior aspect of the talus, from the lateral malleolar region. The patient had a mobile foot type, with excessive range of rearfoot pronation. He also had a leg-length discrepancy, of three-eighths of an inch. Foot and ankle radiographs revealed an area of increased linear density through the neck of the left talus that indicated a healing stress fracture. An isotope bone scan showed increased uptake in the region of the left talus. The patient was treated by way of rest, a below-knee walking cast, and nonsteroidal anti-inflammatory medication. Six weeks later, the cast was removed and six weeks of rehabilitative therapy was prescribed. The patient gradually increased his activity, and eleven months after he had presented, he competed in his first race.

Motto[3] describes the case of a 52-year-old, male competitive-tennis player who presented having had 27 months of ankle pain. When the patient was examined, his subtalar joint mobility was restricted, and both posterior talar compression and hopping on the affected foot were painful. He was at first treated by way of local corticosteroid injections into the sinus tarsi. A CT scan clearly showed a stress fracture involving the lateral process of the talus that extended to the subtalar joint. The talus was explored surgically, and evidence of healing was found at the fracture site. Postoperatively, the patient was allowed to undertake full weightbearing as tolerated. Although the patient improved symptomatically over six months, his subtalar joint range of movement remained restricted. In a repeat CT scan, healing was confirmed, and although the patient was more comfortable during running, he remained unable to play tennis.

Black and Ehlert[4] report the case of a 28-year-old, male orthopedic-surgery resident who had been jogging approximately 60 kilometers per week. The patient presented with a fifteen month history of pain in the region of the lateral aspect of the ankle. His physical examination was unremarkable, and plain radiographs did not show an abnormality. A CT scan revealed an incomplete fracture of the lateral process of the talus that communicated with the subtalar joint. A bone scan revealed focal area of increased uptake in the region of the lateral process.

Although a non-weightbearing below-knee cast was at first proposed as treatment, in keeping with his profession the patient refused immobilization and instead chose to discontinue most athletics activity for three months. He then gradually resumed jogging to a self-imposed maximum of 32 kilometers per week. After two years of follow-up, he was able to participate with occasional discomfort in all the athletics activities he had undertaken before the onset of pain. A repeat CT scan revealed no change in the fracture's appearance. The researchers state that their patient had increased supination of the foot, particularly while running, and that this probably predisposed him to development of a stress fracture. Shelton and Pedowitz[6] describe a concentration of forces of the lateral process of the talus in the supinated foot.

Bradshaw *et al.*[5] present four cases of lateral talar body stress fracture for which all the patients clinically presented with lateral ankle pain of gradual onset. All four patients had typical symptoms and signs of severe sinus tarsi syndrome. A plain radiograph failed to reveal the fracture in any of the four cases, and an isotope bone scan was conducted that showed a typical appearance in all the cases (Fig. 10.1). The fracture was clearly shown on a CT scan in all four cases (Fig. 10.2). Because this type of stress fracture extends into the subtalar joint, this may explain why the condition was originally mistaken for sinus tarsi syndrome. The researchers recommended a six-week period of non-weightbearing rest, followed by a gradual

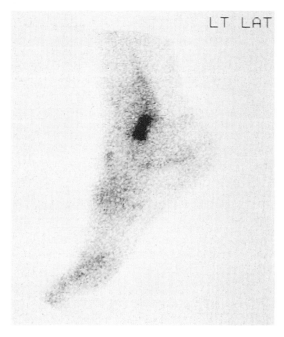

Fig. 10.1
The isotope bone scan appearance of a talar stress fracture.

and supervised rehabilitation program, as the treatment of choice for the four stress fractures.

The researchers postulate that the talar stress fracture's mechanism of development is that in the presence of excessive subtalar pronation and plantar flexion, the lateral process of the calcaneus impinges on the concave posterolateral corner of the talus. All four patients in the series had bilateral increased subtalar pronation. It was believed that correction of the pronation by way of use of orthoses was an important component of the treatment.

Our own recent experience has shown that surgical excision of the lateral process produces good results.

The calcaneus

Calcaneal stress fractures were originally described among the military, and are seen

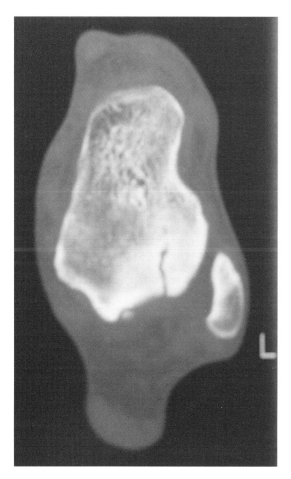

Fig. 10.2
The CT-scan appearance of a talar stress fracture.

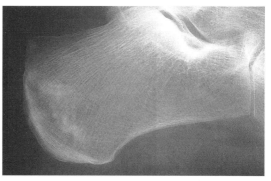

Fig. 10.3
The plain radiograph appearance of a calcaneus stress fracture.

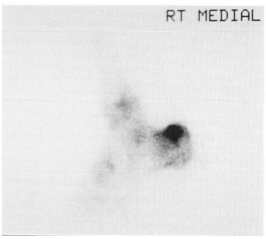

Fig. 10.4
The isotope bone scan appearance of a calcaneus stress fracture.

among runners, ballet dancers, and jumpers. Patients present with a history of insidious onset of heel pain that is aggravated by weightbearing activities, especially running. When the patient is examined, there may be localized tenderness over the medial or lateral aspects of the calcaneus, and pain can be elicited by squeezing the calcaneus from both sides simultaneously. The most common stress-fracture site is the upper posterior margin of the os calcis, just anterior to the apophyseal plate and at right angles to the normal trabecular pattern. The other common site is adjacent to the medial tuberosity, at the point where calcaneal spurs occur.[7]

Plain radiography may show a typical sclerotic appearance that on a lateral X-ray is parallel to the posterior margin of the calcaneus (Fig. 10.3). An isotope bone scan will show a focal area of increased uptake (Fig. 10.4).

Treatment consists of reduction of activity. Non-weightbearing on crutches may be briefly required for pain relief. When the patient is pain free and there is no local tenderness, he or she can commence a program of gradually increased weightbearing over six to eight weeks. Also, he or she should use soft heel pads, undertake joint mobilization, and undertake stretching of the calf muscles and plantar fascia. He or she may also have to use orthoses in order to control excessive pronation.

The cuboid

Very few cases of stress fracture of the cuboid bone are described, and only one of this type of fracture is reported in an athlete.[8] In that case, a twenty-year-old international-level gymnast presented one week after the gradual onset of left-foot pain. The pain affected the lateral aspect of the foot, and was exacerbated by weightbearing, hopping, and resisted plantar flexion. An isotope bone scan revealed abnormal uptake within the left cuboid, and a CT scan (Fig. 10.5) showed a minimally displaced fracture through the medial aspect of the proximal cuboid that had a mainly vertical component. Non-weightbearing on crutches for four weeks was prescribed, followed by progressive weightbearing and reintegration of gymnastic exercises. The patient's recovery over six weeks was good, and there were no more complaints apart from mild pain experienced during specific tumbling exercises. Two months after the fracture had occurred, the athlete resumed normal activity.

The researchers postulate that two factors may be involved in this condition's etiology: chronic repetitive loading, and previous acute trauma (an ankle sprain suffered two years previously).

Hermel and Gershon-Cohen[9] postulate a mechanism known as the 'nut in the nutcracker' that corresponds to a compression of the cuboid

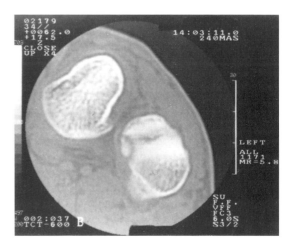

Fig. 10.5
The CT-scan appearance of a cuboid stress fracture.

bone between the calcaneus and the base of the fourth and fifth metatarsals when exaggerated plantar flexion is undertaken. Jahn and Freund[10] describe a similar mechanism that is combined with forefoot inversion.

The cuneiform bones

A small number of stress fractures of the cuneiform bones are reported among military subjects.[11–13] A stress fracture of the lateral cuneiform bone in a basketballer,[14] a stress fracture of the intermediate (or second) cuneiform bone in a triathlete,[15] and a stress fracture of the medial (or first) cuneiform bone in a recreational runner[16] are described.

Khan *et al.*[16] describe a 41-year-old recreational runner who developed intense medial mid-foot pain during a run. The pain persisted despite the patient's six weeks of rest. Examination revealed tenderness over the medial aspect of the medial cuneiform bone, the navicular-cuneiform joint, and the navicular bone distally. When the patient was observed walking, excessive pronation of the subtalar joint was revealed. Although plain radiographs of the foot were normal, an isotope bone scan showed a focal area of increased uptake in the region of the medial cuneiform. A CT scan revealed a zone of sclerosis on the lateral border of the medial cuneiform representing endosteal callus formation (Fig. 10.6). The patient was treated by way of weightbearing rest, and after a period of twelve weeks became pain free when walking. He returned to running over a four-week period, and subsequently increased his running distance to greater than that of his pre-injury level.

Creighton *et al.*[15] report a stress fracture of the intermediate (middle) cuneiform bone in a 55-year-old triathlete who presented having had four months of pain along the dorsum of the left mid foot. An isotope bone scan and a CT scan revealed a fracture in the middle cuneiform bone. Following seven months of 'a host of conservative means of treatment', intraosseous decompression was undertaken in which a Kirschner wire was used to drill three holes in the dorsal surface of the middle cuneiform. Postoperatively, the patient commenced running at four months and remained asymptomatic. The researchers propose that in the runner, the middle cuneiform may be subject to increased stress during the propulsive phase, because it is the bone that transmits weight proximally in the medial column. The region's ligamentous and osseous architecture can also produce a mid-foot buckling when the foot is plantarflexed against resistance.

The navicular

Stress fractures of the tarsal navicular bone are reviewed by Khan *et al.*[17] Navicular stress fractures occur in the sagittal plane involving the middle third of the bone (Fig. 10.7). It is believed that the central third of the navicular is especially susceptible to stress fractures and subsequent delayed union, because of the region of bone's relative avascularity.[18,19]

Traditionally, navicular stress fractures have been viewed as being a relatively uncommon type of stress fracture. However, in recent years, various researchers[19–21] have reported series of navicular stress fractures, and have concluded that the fractures are much more common than

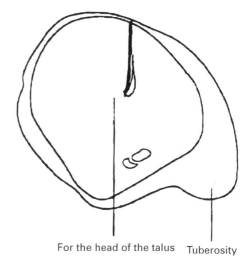

For the head of the talus   Tuberosity

Fig. 10.7
The navicular, showing the plane of the fracture. (Source: Adapted and reproduced, with permission, from Khan KM, Brukner PD, Kearney C *et al.* Tarsal navicular stress fracture in athletes. *Sports Medicine* 1994; 17 (1): 65–76.)

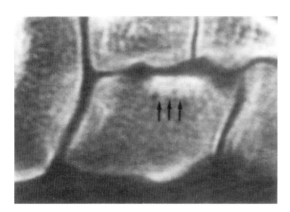

Fig. 10.6
The CT-scan appearance of a medial cuneiform stress fracture.

was earlier thought. Recent stress-fracture series have a high percentage of navicular stress fractures.[22–24] This type of fracture occurs especially in sprinters, and in hurdlers and long jumpers, but also in middle-distance runners. It is also seen in players of football, basketball, racket sports, field hockey, and cricket, and in gymnasts and ballet dancers.

The exact cause of navicular stress fractures is not clear. As is the case with most stress fractures, a combination of overuse and training errors has a significant role in the fractures' development. It is believed that impingement of the navicular occurs between the proximal and distal tarsal bones when the muscles exert bending and compressive forces.[25]

Fitch and colleagues[20] propose that there is a plane of maximum shear stress through the central portion of the navicular (Fig. 10.8). In an unpublished study, our colleagues Agosta and Morarty reveal that of fifteen patients who had navicular stress fracture, thirteen had significantly decreased ankle dorsiflexion. The researchers postulate that this could lead to increased talo-navicular compression. Microangiographic studies of the navicular's blood supply show relative avascularity of the middle third of the bone.[19] A combination of these factors may result in fatigue failure in this portion of the bone, which is consistently the site of stress fractures within the navicular.

The onset of symptoms is usually insidious, and includes increased foot pain after sprinting, jumping, or running.[20] The pain is often vague or ill-defined, especially in the injury's early stages. Most typically, the pain radiates along either the medial aspect of the longitudinal arch or the dorsum of the foot.[19,26] It may also radiate either distally along the first or second ray or laterally toward the cuboid. Neither swelling nor discoloration is usually present. There may be a limp for a short time after exercise is undertaken. The symptoms abate rapidly if the patient rests, and he or she is often able to jog within a week.[20,26,27] Occasionally, there is an acute onset

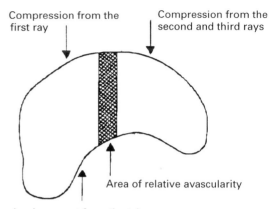

Fig. 10.8
The plane of maximum shear stress through the central portion of the navicular. (Source: Adapted and reproduced, with permission, from Khan KM, Brukner PD, Kearney C *et al.* Tarsal navicular stress fracture in athletes. *Sports Medicine* 1994; 17 (1): 65–76.)

of injury when the patient does not have a history of pain.

When the navicular bone is examined, precise knowledge of the mid foot's anatomy and skillful palpation of the talo-navicular joint are required. Having located the talo-navicular joint while inverting and everting the foot, the examiner palpates the proximal dorsal portion of the navicular. This portion has been described as the 'N-spot',[21,28] and is shown in Fig. 10.9.

Plain radiography has low sensitivity in identification of navicular stress fracture, especially of partial fracture. In their review of the literature about navicular stress fracture, Khan *et al.*[17] report that 86 of the 128 feet that were radiographed had a false-negative result for fracture. Conducting an isotope bone scan is an effective way of revealing increased bony stress in the navicular. All 105 of the isotope scans that were reviewed[17] showed markedly increased focal uptake in the region of the navicular. Of the 105 patients, 82 had previously had a false-negative result when investigated by way of plain radiography. It has been found that plantar

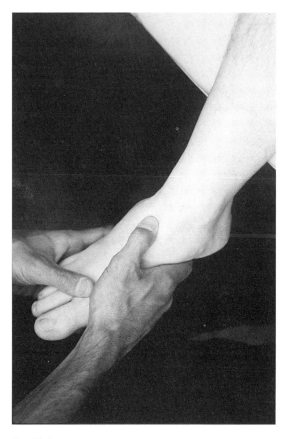

Fig. 10.9
Palpation of the 'N' spot.

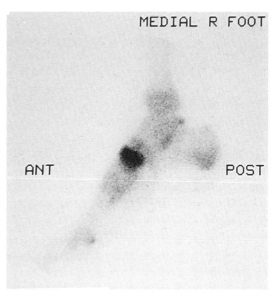

Fig. 10.10
The isotope bone scan appearance of a navicular stress fracture.

views are more useful than the standard frontal, medial, and lateral views.[29] The characteristic appearance of a positive isotope bone scan is that of increased uptake in the entire navicular bone (Fig. 10.10).

A CT scan is valuable for assessing navicular stress fracture. Use of a precise radiologic technique is required for revealing these tiny navicular stress fractures. A bone algorithm must be used and must be oriented through the plane of the talo-navicular joint in order to take contiguous 1.5 millimeter slices (Fig. 10.11).[30] On a CT scan, the appearance of the proximal articular rim of the normal navicular bone is extremely dense and almost sclerotic, and

on true axial images is ringlike (Fig. 10.12). This apparent bone sclerosis may reflect the mechanical load that is normally borne by the relatively small, concave, articular surface of the navicular during weightbearing.[30] Most stress fractures are linear defects, some have associated bone fragments, and others appear as rim defects that do not have a linear component.[30] The typical CT appearance of a navicular stress fracture is shown in Fig. 10.13.

Various treatments are reported for navicular stress fracture. They include simple weightbearing rest, non-weightbearing cast immobilization for two weeks to three months, and surgery. Historically, there has been a high incidence of delayed union and nonunion,[19–21,31] which have in some cases prevented the athletes from returning to their athletics career. In the literature, of the 131 cases in which the outcome was reported, 77 had a satisfactory result whereby the athlete returned to activity with either no or minimal pain after the early treatment was undertaken (Table 10.1).

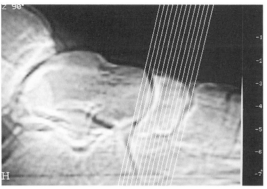

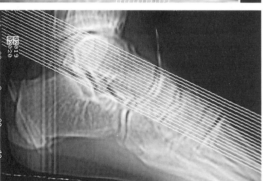

Fig. 10.11
The orientation for a CT scan of the navicular. The broken lines indicate the scan planes and the region to be scanned: **a** Axial scans are obtained with the foot down. The gantry is angled to the plane of the talo-navicular joint. The scans of 1.5 millimeter sections begin just proximal to the navicular articular rim. **b** Coronal scans are obtained with the foot in the anatomic position. The gantry is tilted to the approximate plane of the dorsal surface of the bone. The scans of 3 millimeter sections include the proximal dorsal articular margin of the bone.

For navicular stress fractures, early treatment by way of weightbearing rest has met with a high failure rate. Of forty-five fractures at first treated in this way, only eleven healed, and then only slowly, although without complication.[19–21,31] In the literature, all five cases of refracture were at first treated by way of weightbearing rest. Although decreased activity alone may alleviate the symptoms, it will not enable osteoblastic activity to bridge the fracture site.[32,33]

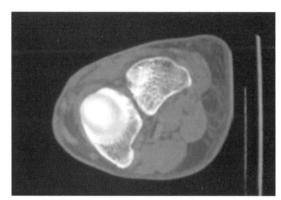

Fig. 10.12
The CT-scan appearance of a normal navicular.

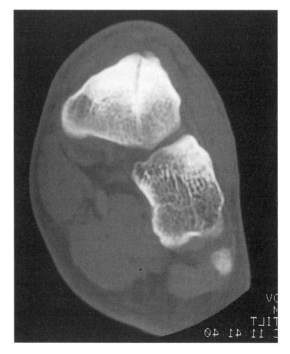

Fig. 10.13
The typical CT-scan appearance of a navicular stress fracture.

Table 10.1 A summary of the successful outcomes of early treatment published in reports about navicular stress fractures

Treatment	Torg et al. (1982)	Fitch et al. (1989)	Khan et al. (1992)	Others*	Total* (%)
Weightbearing rest	2/9	–	9/34	0/2	11/45 (24)
Surgery	2/2	12/15*	5/6	2/3	21/26 (81)
Non-weightbearing cast (more than six weeks)	9/9	–	19/22	4/5	32/36 (89)
Other treatment	–	–	13/24	–	13/24 (54)

*Note: * Total follow-up number lower than total number of cases described.*
(Source: Adapted and reproduced, with permission, from Khan KM, Brukner PD, Kearney C et al. Tarsal navicular stress fractures in athletes. Sports Medicine *1994; 17 (1): 65–76.)*

By contrast, navicular stress fractures that are treated by way of non-weightbearing cast immobilization have excellent results. Thirty-two of thirty-six patients were asymptomatic after treatment was undertaken. Six patients who had a complete navicular stress fracture and who were at first treated by way of non-weightbearing cast immobilization recovered uneventfully.[19,21] Furthermore, of ten patients who were at first treated by way of weightbearing rest and who continued to have symptoms and were subsequently treated by way of non-weightbearing cast immobilization, nine fully recovered.[19,21] One patient who had internal fixation as the first treatment but who had persistent symptoms, also fully recovered by way of subsequent non-weightbearing cast immobilization.

Among the reported cases, of twenty-seven fractures that were complicated by either delayed union or displacement of fragments, twenty-two were successfully treated by way of surgery. Surgical methods include internal fixation, or curettage and grafting. At operation, the fracture is difficult to visualize unless there is wide separation of the fragments, because the dorsal surface of the navicular bone is rarely disrupted. It is frequently necessary to open the talo-navicular joint and to separate the articular surfaces by way of traction.[20] According to

another report, a Kirschner wire was vertically inserted from above in the estimated fracture site, and during the operation, CT scanning was used in order to ascertain the wire's position relative to the fracture and to thereby localize the fracture.[33] In most cases, the postoperative treatment involved six weeks' non-weightbearing either with or without cast immobilization.

For the patient who presents with persistent mid-foot pain that is aggravated by activity and who has a clinical finding of tenderness at the 'N' spot, investigation by way of radionuclide scan is usually required, because radiography's sensitivity for navicular stress fracture is extremely low. If the radionuclide scan shows focal uptake in the navicular bone, a fine-slice CT scan is required in the plane of the talo-navicular joint in order to differentiate between a stress fracture and a stress reaction, because management of one would differ from that of the other.[21] A navicular stress reaction (a positive isotope bone scan and a negative CT scan) would be treated by way of weightbearing rest and close observation.

A management algorithm for navicular stress fracture is shown in Fig. 10.14.

After either partial or complete navicular stress fracture has been diagnosed by way of either plain radiography or a CT scan, the patient must be treated by way of *strict* non-

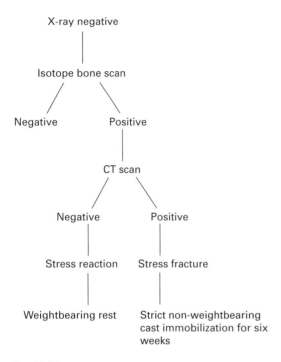

Fig. 10.14
A management algorithm for navicular stress fracture.

weightbearing cast immobilization for a least six weeks. Because waterproof underwrap and casting material are now available, it is possible for patients to shower, to swim, or to run in the water (see Chapter 5) while casted. Even complete fractures in which the segments have apparently separated should be treated in this way at first.

Patients should be reviewed three weeks after they have been casted. The review provides an opportunity to assess the state of the cast, to re-emphasize the importance of strict non-weightbearing, and to explain the rehabilitation program that is to commence when the cast is removed. The cast should be removed after six weeks, and the healing should be assessed clinically. The radiologic appearance after six weeks of cast immobilization is not a useful indicator of healing, so X-ray, isotope bone scan and CT scan are not indicated at that stage.[16]

Athletes often feel some diffuse foot pain and paresthesia when they first walk after having non-weightbearing cast immobilization. However, the pain usually differs from the pain they had when they presented, and it diminishes when they undertake passive joint mobilization and weightbearing activity. It is believed that the pain is the result of joint stiffness of the talo-crural, subtalar and mid-tarsal joints,[34] because of the cast immobilization. As long as the navicular bone is not tender, the pain is not contraindicated in weightbearing rehabilitation.

If the fracture is clinically healed (no tenderness is present at the 'N' spot), a six-week program of rehabilitation supervised by a sports physiotherapist is recommended. The program includes a graduated return to activity, joint mobilization, soft-tissue massage, and muscle strengthening. If tenderness remains over the 'N' spot, Khan *et al.*[16] recommend the patient have two more weeks' non-weightbearing in a cast, that the cast then be removed, and that the patient undergo rehabilitation.

The following rehabilitation program is recommended.[16] For the first two weeks of weightbearing, the patient is allowed to undertake normal activities of daily living, swimming, and water running. After this period, the 'N' spot is reassessed, and if there is no increase in tenderness, the athlete may begin jogging on grass for five minutes on alternate days. After three or four of these sessions, the jogging time can be increased to ten minutes. The athlete is reassessed after two weeks of jogging. If the 'N' spot is not tender, the athlete can begin to undertake 'run-throughs' (faster running, over 50 to 80 meters) and on alternate days walk recovery. The speed is gradually increased from half to three-quarters of maximum speed over another two weeks. After a total of six weeks' rehabilitation, the athlete is reassessed, and if the 'N' spot is not tender, he or she is allowed to continue to gradually return to full training.

After the cast is removed, the associated stiffness of the talo-crural, subtalar and mid-tarsal joints should be treated by way of passive joint mobilization.[28] Often, there will also be soft-tissue tightness, especially in the tibialis posterior and soleus muscles, which should be treated by way of techniques for active stretching and soft-tissue massage, including myofascial release.[28,35] Muscle weakness that results from atrophy during the non-weightbearing period has to be corrected by way of a graded strengthening program before the athlete is allowed to fully resume activity.

It has been shown that when this treatment regimen is followed, almost all navicular stress fractures progress to clinical union. If after strict adherence to the treatment program there is no evidence of clinical healing, surgery should be undertaken. Screw fixation is the recommended surgical method. Some surgeons also use bone grafting in cases of established nonunion. A small fragment (or ossicle) may occasionally be present at the dorsal surface. This may act as a wedge, and the practitioner should consider surgically removing it.

As is the case with any overuse injury, the possibility that abnormal biomechanics contributed should be assessed. Although clinical researchers have not yet isolated any specific biomechanic abnormality that is common to all athletes who have a navicular stress fracture, we believe that any significant biomechanic abnormality (for example excessive subtalar joint pronation) should be corrected by way of orthotics, and that any joint stiffness (for example decreased ankle dorsiflexion) should be treated by way of joint mobilization.

An accessory navicular bone is occasionally present, and the patient may become symptomatic. Although this type of patient presents with symptoms similar to those of the patient who has a navicular stress fracture, his or her tenderness is maximal over tuberosity of the navicular, not over the 'N' spot. An X-ray reveals that an accessory navicular is present, and an isotope bone scan shows increased uptake in the region of the accessory navicular rather than in the whole bone. A CT scan reveals that a pseudoarticulation is present between the accessory and the navicular. This scenario represents a stress reaction, and the patient should be treated by way of an orthotic if excessive foot pronation exists, and by way of weightbearing rest.

Navicular stress fractures are much more common than was previously thought, and aggressive non-weightbearing cast immobilization is required as the first line of treatment. For patients who are treated in this way, the healing rate is high.

The metatarsals: general

In most stress-fracture series, the metatarsal bones are the second-most common fracture site, after the tibia. Metatarsal stress fracture was first described by Briethaupt,[36] who called the condition *fussgeschwulst*, which means 'traumatic inflammation of the tendon sheaths'. The condition, which was common among soldiers, eventually became known as 'march foot' and later as 'march fracture'.

This type of fracture is especially prevalent among distance runners and ballet dancers. Although management of most metatarsal stress fractures is relatively straightforward, the two major exceptions are fracture of the base of the second metatarsal and fracture of the diaphysis of the fifth metatarsal. Both of these fractures will be considered separately.

The most common site of metatarsal stress fracture is the neck of the second metatarsal. One reason for this may be that because in the pronating foot the first ray is dorsiflexed, the second metatarsal is subjected to greater load. Because the base of the second metatarsal is firmly fixed in position next to the cuneiform bones, the likelihood of fracture is increased even more. Stress fracture of the second metatarsal is especially common among ballet dancers, who invariably already have a considerable amount of cortical hypertrophy of the second metatarsal.

It has been suggested that the second metatarsal is particularly susceptible to stress fracture in the case of a Morton's foot, in which the first ray is shorter than the second. However, this theory has been challenged by Harris and Beath,[37] as well as by Drez et al.[38] Harris and Beath[37] studied the feet of more than a thousand Canadian soldiers who were undergoing strenuous military training, and they failed to find any disability caused by a short first metatarsal. Drez et al.[38] studied the radiographs of sixty-five patients who had a metatarsal stress fracture, and compared them with the fifty radiographs of a control group of randomly selected people for whom there was no record of foot problems. Statistical analysis of the ratios between the absolute lengths of the first and second metatarsals, and of the ratios between the relative lengths of the first and second metatarsals, revealed no significant differences between the two groups.

The patient who has a metatarsal stress fracture complains of forefoot pain that is aggravated by activity such as running or dancing. Although the pain is not severe at first, it gradually worsens when activity is undertaken. If marked focal tenderness is present, stress fracture is suggested. Metatarsal stress fracture is mainly a clinical diagnosis, and in most cases it is not necessary to image the fracture.

However, presence of a stress fracture may be confirmed by way of X-ray, the appearance of which may vary from that of a displaced fracture or radiolucent line (Fig. 10.15) to that of a more subtle area of focal periosteal thickening (Fig. 10.16). If plain radiography does not confirm that a fracture is present, an isotope bone scan can be conducted.

Treatment consists of rest from the aggravating activity. Progress should be monitored clinically, and the athlete should be allowed to recommence his or her sporting

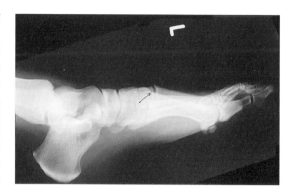

Fig. 10.15
The radiograph appearance of a metatarsal stress fracture.

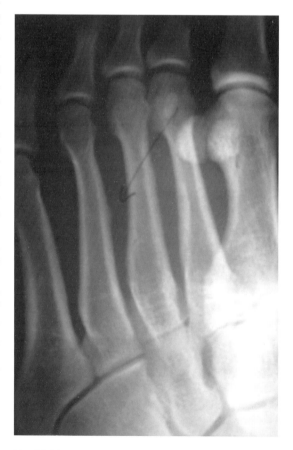

Fig. 10.16
A radiograph that shows periosteal thickening of the metatarsal.

activities when he or she does not experience pain when walking and there is no local tenderness at the fracture site. He or she should have a graduated exercise program in order to return to full training and competition. Any biomechanic abnormality that may be present, especially any instability that is experienced during forefoot weightbearing, should be corrected by way of orthoses.

The second metatarsal: base

Stress fracture of the base of the second metatarsal is described[39–41] among ballet dancers. It was the most common stress-fracture site in a twelve-year study of injuries sustained by members of the Australian Ballet (Crichton, personal communication). All the dancers presented with mid-foot pain that was worse *en pointe* and when jumps were undertaken. Clinically, it was impossible to differentiate between the dancers who had traumatic synovitis of the second tarso-metatarsal joint (Lisfranc's joint) and stress fracture of the base of the second metatarsal.

Micheli *et al.*[39] review the cases of four female ballet dancers, all of whom presented with a lengthy history of pain over the dorsum of the mid foot that was localized to the region of the base of the second metatarsal. The pain was aggravated when the dancer was in the full *en pointe* position. The researchers advocate that the first assessment should include not only anteroposterior and lateral radiographs of the foot but two oblique radiographs. One of their patients required surgical resection because of persistent nonunion of a necrotic fracture fragment. The other three patients healed by way of varying lengths of partial and non-weightbearing cast immobilization.

For the eight Australian Ballet dancers who presented with a similar clinical picture,[40] no fracture line was seen on the plain radiograph. The eight patients were then examined by way of

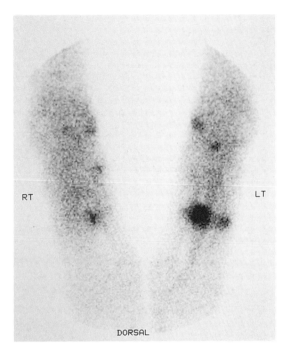

Fig. 10.17
The isotope bone scan appearance of a stress fracture of the second metatarsal.

scintigraphy, which showed increased uptake of isotope that was localized to the area of the second tarso-metatarsal articulation (Fig. 10.17). The eight patients were examined by way of MRI, and in six of them a bone stress reaction was revealed at the base of the second metatarsal. On the T1-weighted images, evidence of bone stress reaction is decreased signal from the medulla. Of the six patients, the MRI of four also showed a low signal line from cortex to cortex, which indicated a fracture line (Fig. 10.18).

For the two ballerinas who had a normal MRI, traumatic synovitis was diagnosed by exclusion. For the four patients for whom a fracture line was revealed by way of MRI, each fracture was shown to run with a similar obliquity across the base of the second metatarsal. In the sagittal plane, the fracture extended obliquely superoposteriorly from the inferior cortical

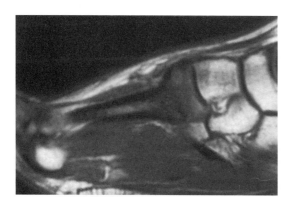

Fig. 10.18
The MRI appearance of a stress fracture of the second metatarsal.

margin of the second-metatarsal base. Of the six patients who had stress fracture, three followed the researchers' advice to rest from all dancing until they were no longer tender over the base of the second metatarsal. This rest was followed by a gradual return to dancing, and by avoidance of jumps, *en pointe* work and other painful movements in the early period. The three dancers required rest for only six to eight weeks, and had another month of gradually increased activity until they fully resumed dancing. The dancers who continued to dance even in a modified way had a prolonged period of time until full recovery, and one of them had incomplete union of the fracture. The two patients who were diagnosed as having traumatic synovitis were treated by way of two weeks of nonsteroidal anti-inflammatory medication, along with passive mobilization of the second tarso-metatarsal articulation and temporary reduction of jumping and performing in the *en pointe* position. Despite the fact they continued to dance, both the patients were symptom free within six weeks, and remained so.

From this series, it would seem that if this type of stress fracture is recognized early and treated appropriately, healing should result. It would also seem that in this type of stress fracture, MRI is the best form of imaging for differentiating between the two possible diagnoses, because the

isotope bone scan is not specific and the CT scan will not image a stress reaction.

O'Malley *et al.*[41] reviewed fifty-one professional dancers who had sixty-four stress fractures of the base of the second metatarsal. The clinical presentation was insidious onset of mid-foot pain at an average of 2.5 weeks before the patient sought medical care. For all the patients, physical examination revealed tenderness either at the base of the first web space or on the proximal portion of the second metatarsal. The pain was exacerbated by the relevé maneuver (the dancer is up on the balls of his or her feet). The first radiographs of the foot were positive for nineteen patients, questionable for three patients, and negative for forty-two patients. The standard foot series of radiographs was supplemented with a special posterior–anterior (PA) view ('the dancer's view') of the foot in an attempt to eliminate overlap of the joints at the base of the second metatarsal, which is common in the cavus foot that is frequently found in ballet dancers. This X-ray is taken by using the same technique as for a standard AP foot radiograph, except that the foot is positioned 'upside down' whereby the dorsum of the foot is against the cassette (Fig. 10.19).

Treatment consisted of wearing a short-leg walking cast for six patients, and wearing a wooden shoe and having symptomatic treatment for the others. At follow-up, 14% of the patients continued to occasionally have either pain or stiffness in the mid foot while dancing. The patients returned to performing at an average of 6.2 weeks following diagnosis. None of them required bone grafting for persistent symptoms. Eight refractures occurred at the same site at an average of 4.3 years, and all of them healed by way of conservative care.

The etiology of this fracture is uncertain. Hamilton[42] suggests that the factors that predispose a person to this type of stress fracture include amenorrhea, anorexia nervosa, Morton's foot, a cavus foot, and anterior ankle impingement. In the Australian Ballet study,

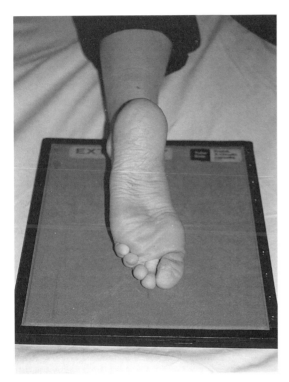

Fig. 10.19
The positioning for a PA radiograph of the foot.

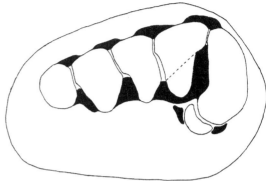

Fig. 10.20
A suggested mechanism of injury for stress fracture of the second metatarsal.

three of the eight dancers (of whom one had traumatic synovitis) did not menstruate, six had a Morton's foot, and of the six, five had a stress fracture. This syndrome has been recognized only among female ballet dancers, which suggests that the *en pointe* position is the precipitating factor. Hamilton[42] suggests the syndrome has a biomechanic cause, and describes the middle cuneiform as being the keystone of the transverse arch of the mid foot that holds the arch rigid. The base of the second metatarsal is countersunk into the bony arch of this keystone's distal bony arch, and is consequently held rigid.

Harrington *et al.*[40] state that the fracture's orientation seemed to be explicable mainly on anatomic grounds. The interosseous ligaments between the base of the second metatarsal and the medial cuneiform medially, and between the base of the third metatarsal laterally, firmly hold the plantar part of the base of the second metatarsal. The dorsal part of the base of the second metatarsal is enabled to have more freedom of movement. This is accommodated for by cartilage articulations dorsally with the medial cuneiform and base of the third metatarsal. The small amount of motion that is enabled to occur in the sagittal plane therefore has, as its fulcrum, interosseus attachments. As is the case with many stress-related fractures, the fracture line extends along the edge of fixation. This suggested mechanism of injury is shown in Fig. 10.20.

The *en pointe* position exacerbates these forces that are applied to the base of the second metatarsal. The compressive forces that are applied to the second metatarsal are increased in the case of a Morton's foot. The peroneus longus and tibialis posterior, which are important muscles for maintaining the *en pointe* position, commonly have an attachment to the base of the second metatarsal and thereby offer traction specifically to the immobilized fracture site.

In summary, stress fractures of the base of the second metatarsal are common among female ballet dancers. A plain radiograph that includes a special PA view of the foot, and isotope bone scan, should be used in order to confirm the diagnosis. Most patients will return to dancing after having six weeks of rest and undertaking a graduated activity program.

The fifth metatarsal: proximal

Fractures of the proximal third of the fifth metatarsal have caused considerable confusion among practitioners. In this region, there are three types of fracture: the tuberosity avulsion fracture, the Jones' fracture at the junction of the metaphysis and diaphysis, and the diaphyseal stress fracture (Fig. 10.21).

Previously, the Jones' fracture and the diaphyseal stress fracture were grouped together, and some practitioners continue to describe all fractures of the proximal fifth metatarsal other than the tuberosity avulsion fracture as being 'Jones' fractures'. Although the tuberosity avulsion fracture and the true Jones' fracture are actually acute fractures, they are briefly included in this section in an attempt to clear up the confusion.

This region's anatomy has been described by Dameron, Torg *et al.*, and Richli and Rosenthal.[43–45] Sir Robert Jones himself[46] emphasized the very strong soft-tissue

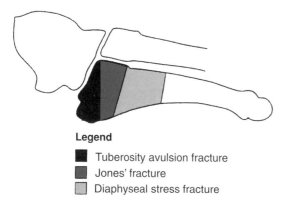

Legend

■ Tuberosity avulsion fracture
■ Jones' fracture
□ Diaphyseal stress fracture

Fig. 10.21
Three sites for fracture of the proximal third of the fifth metatarsal. (Source: Lawrence SR, Botte MJ. Jones' fracture and related fractures of the proximal fifth metatarsal. *Foot and Ankle* 1993; 14 (6): 358–365.)

connections located at the base of the fifth metatarsal and the strong connection between this metatarsal and the adjacent metatarsal and cuboid bones.

Stewart[47] suggests that up to seven structures insert on the proximal fifth metatarsal. Although the joint capsule is probably the strongest structure, the peroneus brevis and tertius, the abductor digiti minimi, the flexor digiti minimi, and the interosseous muscles all insert in this region. There is also a band of plantar fascia that inserts in the most proximal tip of the fifth metatarsal. Richli and Rosenthal[45] show that the lateral cord of plantar fascia attaches proximally to the other tendons. They also show that the force that is applied to this structure results in a transverse fracture through the tuberosity of the metatarsal posterior to most of the peroneus brevis insertion. An athlete whose sport involves repetitive pivoting inward and outward while he or she is weightbearing across the ball of the foot may be especially susceptible to problems in this area.[48]

The base of the fifth metatarsal consists mostly of cancellous bone with extremely thin cortices. Because it is well vascularized, the region heals promptly and predictably. However, at the junction of the proximal metaphysis and diaphysis, the cortex thickens considerably and the medullary canal narrows, whereby a transition is made from mostly cancellous to relatively avascular cortical bone. In runners, the cortices can thicken even more and thereby cause the already poor blood supply to be more diminished. This poor vascularity retards the area's bone healing.[49,50]

The most common fracture that is seen is a simple avulsion fracture of the tuberosity at the base of the fifth metatarsal. It has always been believed that this was caused by contraction of the peroneus brevis tendon as a result of an acute inversion injury; however, more recently, the lateral band of the plantar aponeurosis has been implicated[45] (Fig. 10.22). This is usually an uncomplicated type of fracture that usually

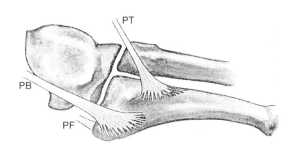

Fig. 10.22
Muscle attachments to the base of the fifth metatarsal. (Source: Lawrence SR, Botte MJ. Jones' fracture and related fractures of the proximal fifth metatarsal. *Foot and Ankle* 1993; 14 (6): 358–365.) PB = Peroneus brevis; PF = Plantar fascia; PT = Peroneus tertius.

heals well if the patient has a short period of immobilization for pain relief.

Sir Robert Jones[46] describes an acute transverse fracture at the junction of the diaphysis and metaphysis that he sustained while dancing around a tent pole at a military party. The Jones' fracture is a transverse fracture at the junction of the diaphysis and metaphysis, in the region up to 1.5 centimeters from the tuberosity. Although it may involve the articular facet between the fourth and fifth metatarsals, it does not extend distal to this articulation. Taking an oblique radiograph is essential for evaluating the fracture's precise location in relation to the facet. In order to avoid confusion, the term 'Jones' fracture' should be reserved for referring to acute fractures located in this precise region.

The Jones' fracture occurs when the ankle is plantar flexed and a strong adduction force is applied to the forefoot. This type of fracture occurs most frequently among football, basketball and tennis players. Because of the poor blood supply, Jones' fractures are prone to delayed union and nonunion if treatment is less than optimal.

The acute, nondisplaced Jones' fracture should be treated by way of non-weightbearing immobilization for four weeks, followed by a walking cast for another four weeks. Most fractures will heal if this regimen is followed. However, the practitioner should consider treating professional athletes aggressively by way of percutaneous intramedullary screw fixation.[43,51–53] People who show inadequate clinical evidence of healing after the period of cast immobilization could, depending on the person, have continued cast immobilization, continued protection, or surgical intervention. The clinician should rely on clinical evidence of healing, because the radiographic appearance of healing lags well behind. Although Jones' fractures are typically undisplaced, the occasional displaced fracture should be treated by way of open reduction and internal fixation.

The recommended surgical technique involves percutaneous insertion of a cannulated screw that is placed longitudinally down the intramedullary canal. Active patients typically recover from the surgery quickly, bear weight within days, begin aerobic activities such as cycling within the first week, and return to full activity in four to eight weeks. The screw is well tolerated, and can remain *in situ*.

Stress fractures of the diaphyseal shaft of the fifth metatarsal occur in the proximal 1.5 centimeters of the shaft. Although many studies of this fracture are published in the literature,[43,51,54–56] most of them also include the true Jones' fracture in this group. Torg *et al.*[44] describe three main subtypes of the diaphyseal stress fracture: acute (or early), delayed union, and nonunion.

The first (Torg Type 1) subtype is an 'acute' fracture whereby the patient has no history of pain in the region of the fracture. What Torg *et al.*[44] describe as 'acute' was an 'early' stress fracture with periosteal reaction that represents an attempt to heal an incomplete fracture. An X-ray confirms presence of periosteal reaction, and reveals no medullary sclerosis (Fig. 10.23). These acute fractures have a good prognosis provided they are treated by way of immobilization in a short-leg, non-weightbearing cast. We recommend that the patient at first

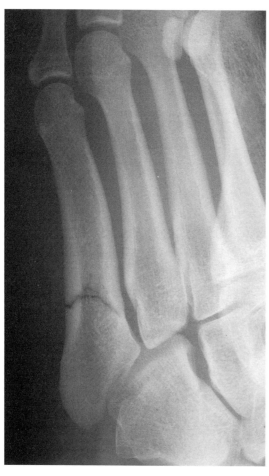

Fig. 10.23
A plain radiograph that shows a Torg Type 1 fracture.

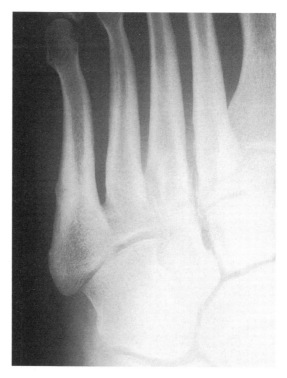

Fig. 10.24
A plain radiograph that shows a Torg Type 2 fracture.

be placed in a cast for six weeks, and that at the time of removal his or her healing be assessed both clinically and radiologically. It may be necessary to immobilize the foot for another period, of up to four weeks. Nonunion may occasionally occur, and can be treated surgically.

For a diaphyseal fracture, the most common presentation is an acute presentation of a stress fracture (Torg Type 2). Although the patient at first presents with what seems to be an acute fracture, when questioned he or she describes a variable period of pain when activity is

undertaken in the region of the fracture. An X-ray reveals a fracture line and, depending on the symptoms' duration, may reveal some evidence of cortical thickening and medullary sclerosis (Fig. 10.24). This type of fracture is prone to delayed union and nonunion, although most of the fractures will eventually heal if conservatively managed. However, most patients are reluctant to have a prolonged period of time in a cast, and for these cases of acute presentation of a diaphyseal stress fracture, we recommend surgical management by way of percutaneous screw fixation.

For a diaphyseal stress fracture, the third type of presentation is a presentation whereby there is an established nonunion radiographically, with complete intramedullary obliteration (Torg Type 3) (Fig. 10.25). These patients should be treated

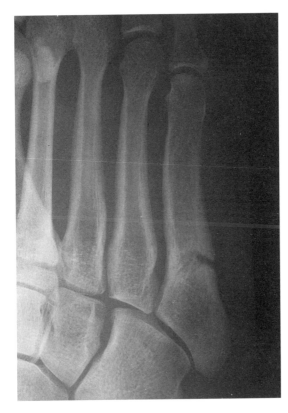

Fig. 10.25
A plain radiograph that shows a Torg Type 3 fracture.

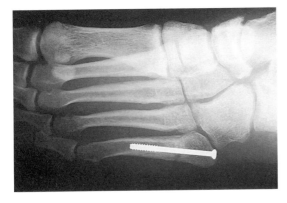

Fig. 10.26
A screw *in situ.*

by way of either screw fixation (Fig. 10.26) or bone grafting. Progressive weightbearing is initiated at two weeks after screw fixation in a hard-sole shoe, and return to running is as early as seven weeks.[51] Because bone grafting requires at least twelve weeks for bony healing, weightbearing activities are delayed.[57]

The diaphyseal stress fracture of the fifth metatarsal is one of the small group of stress fractures for which early recognition and aggressive treatment are required in order to maximize the possibility of complete healing.

The sesamoids

The term 'sesamoid' is derived from the Greek word *sesamum*, because the bones resemble the seeds of the plant *Sesamum indicum* that was used as a purgative by the Ancient Greeks.[58] The Ancient Arabs believed that the great-toe sesamoids had magical properties. In 400 AD, Ushaia inspected many graves in his search for the seat of the soul. He noted that the sesamoids were the best preserved of all the bones. He therefore decided that they were the repository, or storehouse, for the soul, and that on judgement day they would be watered with celestial dew, whereupon the body would be reconstituted around them.

The medial and lateral sesamoid bones at the first metatarso-phalangeal (MTP) joint have a number of functions. They act to increase the mechanical advantage of the flexor hallucis brevis tendon, they act to stabilize the first MTP joint in association with the plantar plate capsule, they act to protect the flexor hallucis longus tendon, and they absorb weightbearing stress on the medial forefoot. They may be injured in a number of ways, including traumatic fracture, stress fracture, and sprain of a bipartite sesamoid. Inflammatory changes and osteonecrosis around the sesamoid and the tendon are collectively known as sesamoiditis. The medial sesamoid is the bone that is affected most often.

Van Hal *et al.*[59] first described sesamoid stress fractures. In the researchers' series, four patients (one male and three females, whose mean age was twenty-one years) experienced insidious onset of pain in the area of their first MTP joint during and/or after athletics activity. They had tenderness to palpation, and pain when their first MTP joint was forcibly dorsiflexed. In all four cases, the stress fracture was revealed by way of plain radiography, although in three of the cases previous radiographs had failed to reveal the fracture. The bone scan was also positive in all four cases.

In this series, two of the stress fractures were in the medial sesamoid, and two in the lateral. None of the four patients had healing of their fracture by way of six weeks of casting and/or four to six months of inactivity. All four eventually had their sesamoid excised. After the surgery, they were placed in a short-leg cast for three weeks. At that point, the cast was removed and the patients were encouraged to increase their activity as tolerated. They returned to their prefracture activities without symptoms in an average of ten weeks after surgery, and remained symptom free.

Hulkko *et al.*[60] describe fifteen cases of stress fracture of the sesamoid bones among athletes. Eight of the fractures were located in the medial, six in the lateral, and one in both sesamoids. Ten of the patients were treated conservatively by way of avoiding excessive physical activity and wearing better training shoes. In five cases, the fragmented sesamoid bone was surgically excised. There were no complications in the series, and the athletes could start gradually training six to eight weeks after the operation. Three of the conservatively treated athletes had mild symptoms during intensive training, and the other seven had a good end result.

Clinically, it is difficult to differentiate between a sesamoid stress fracture and other causes of sesamoid pain. The patient complains of pain when forefoot weightbearing is undertaken, and will often walk with his or her weight laterally

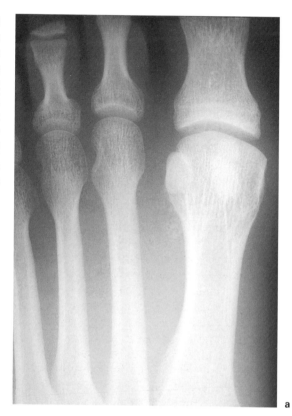

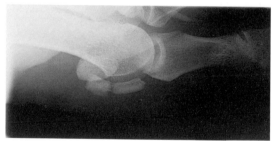

Fig. 10.27
The sesamoids: **a** Stress fracture; **b** Bipartite sesamoid.

in order to compensate. When he or she is examined, there is marked tenderness and occasionally swelling in the region of the sesamoid. An X-ray may reveal presence of a stress fracture, but may not distinguish it from bipartite or multipartite sesamoid bones (Fig. 10.27).

Bilateral foot radiographs are of little value, because 75% of people who have multipartite sesamoids have this variation bilaterally.[61–63] The radiologic signs of sesamoid stress fracture include a transverse fracture line (or possibly two lines) that has jagged margins and sharp corners. Compared with the bone's contours, the margins are more osteoporotic. The fracture line widens during the follow-up, and the margins become smoother. The bone can sometimes be splintered into several fragments. Callus formation may be seen on later radiographs.

An isotope bone scan should be conducted if a stress fracture is suspected but the radiograph is negative. Biedert[64] advocates use of an isotope bone scan and of a subsequent CT scan in order to diagnose sesamoid stress fracture. He states that it is essential that longitudinal scans be conducted. Burton and Amaker[65] report a case in which they used MRI in order to diagnose a stress fracture of the great-toe sesamoid. They describe the sesamoid's appearance as being flattened, fragmented, and hypointense on T1- and T2-weighted images.

Stress fractures of the sesamoid bones are prone to nonunion, and may require an extended period of non-weightbearing. Davis and Alexander[66] recommend casting for six weeks as the first treatment. If at that point clinical or radiographic healing is incomplete, recasting is recommended. Sesamoidectomy is then indicated for patients who have persistent symptoms despite having appropriate conservative management.

McBryde and Anderson[67] recommend casting with full-length platform support, and specific prevention of dorsiflexion. They advocate bone grafting for delayed union and nonunion, although selected partial or complete excision may be necessary.

We recommend that this type of stress fracture be treated in a non-weightbearing cast for six weeks. After the cast is removed, gradual weightbearing can be commenced when bony tenderness is no longer present. Padding is used

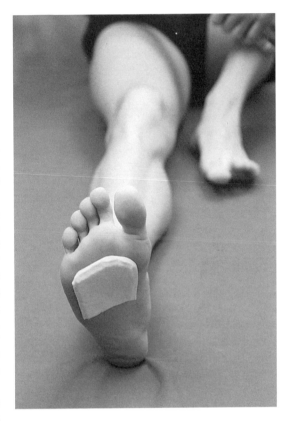

Fig. 10.28
Padding for distributing weight away from the sesamoid bone.

in order to distribute the weight away from the sesamoid bone (Fig. 10.28). If nonunion occurs, or if the bone is splintered into a number of fragments, excision is recommended. The practitioner should also consider partial excision if the distal fragment is smaller in association with a reconstruction and attachment of the flexor hallucis brevis tendon.

The great toe

Stress fractures of the proximal phalanx of the great toe are reported among adolescent athletes.[68,69]

Yokoe and Mannoji[68] report three cases of stress fracture of the proximal phalanx of the great toe in a sprinter, a *Kendo* (Japanese fencing) player, and a rugby-football player. The patients were twelve, sixteen and twenty-one years old, respectively. In all three cases, a definite fracture was revealed at the medial base of the proximal phalanx of the great toe. All three patients had a marked hallux valgus. The researchers postulate that the extensor hallucis longus tendon and the adductor hallucis tendon have a bow-stringing effect on the hallux valgus, and that during activity, the extensor hallucis longus tendon has a continuous bow-stringing effect on the big toe and the medial collateral ligament, thereby causing an avulsion-type stress fracture of the proximal phalanx of the great toe.

When an activity such as running or jumping is undertaken, vertical ground-reaction forces can be several times the person's body weight.[70] Intense truncation forces as a result of the windlass action of the plantar aponeurosis and of muscle action,[71–74] as well as axial compressive forces,[70,72] are repeatedly exerted on the basal portion of the proximal phalanx.

Shiraishi *et al.*[69] also report three cases of stress fracture of the proximal phalanx of the great toe. The fractures occurred in a twelve-year-old volleyball player, a seventeen-year-old female long-distance runner, and a twelve-year-old soccer player. Of the three cases, only one was associated with hallux valgus. Although one patient healed successfully after having a month of relative rest, one of the other patients continued to train, and the fracture proceeded to nonunion.

The recommended treatment is four to six weeks' avoidance of the aggravating activity, and gradual resumption of training. In our experience, this type of fracture requires eight to ten weeks of gradual resumption of full activity.

SUMMARY

- The patient who has a stress fracture of the lateral body of the talus presents as having a sinus tarsi syndrome, and requires either immobilization or excision.
- Navicular stress fractures are extremely common among runners and jumpers.
- The patient who has a navicular stress fracture presents with vague foot pain, and is tender over his or her dorsal aspect.
- Navicular stress fractures require strict non-weightbearing cast immobilization for six weeks, followed by six weeks of supervised rehabilitation.
- Metatarsal stress fractures are commonly seen among the military, athletes, and dancers.
- Some types of metatarsal stress fracture require specific treatment.
- These fractures include those of the base of the second metatarsal and of the diaphysis of the fifth metatarsal.

References

1   MacGlone JJ. Stress fractures of the talus. *Journal of the American Podiatry Association* 1965; 55: 814–817.

2   Campbell G, Warnekros W. Tarsal stress fracture in a long-distance runner: a case report. *Journal of American Podiatric Association* 1983; 72: 532–535.

3   Motto SG. Stress fracture of the lateral process of the talus – a case report. *British Journal of Sports Medicine* 1993; 27 (4): 275–276.

4   Black KP, Ehlert KJ. A stress fracture of the lateral process of the talus in a runner. *Journal of Bone and Joint Surgery* 1994; 76A (3): 441–443.

5   Bradshaw C, Khan K, Brukner P. Stress fracture of the body of the talus in athletes demonstrated with computer tomography. *Clinical Journal of Sport Medicine* 1996; 6 (1): 48–51.

6   Shelton ML, Pedowitz WJ. Injuries to the talus and midfoot. In: Jahss MH, ed. *Disorders of the Foot.* (Volume 2.) Philadelphia: W. B. Saunders, 1982: 1486–1489.

7 Reid D. *Sports Injury Assessment and Rehabilitation*. New York: Churchill Livingstone, 1992.

8 Mahler P, Fricker P. Case report: cuboid stress fracture. *Excel* 1992; 8: 147–148.

9 Hermel MB, Gershon-Cohen J. The nutcracker fracture of the cuboid by indirect violence. *Radiology* 1953; 60: 850–854.

10 Jahn H, Freund KJ. Isolated fractures of the cuboid bone: two case reports with review of the literature. *Journal of Foot Surgery* 1989; 28 (6): 512–515.

11 Gilbert RS, Johnson HA. Stress fractures in military recruits – a review of twelve years' experience. *Military Medicine* 1966; 131: 716–721.

12 Protzman RR, Griffis CG. Stress fractures in men and women undergoing military training. *Journal of Bone and Joint Surgery* 1977; 59-A: 825.

13 Meurman KOA, Elfving S. Stress fracture of the cuneiform bones. *British Journal of Radiology* 1980; 53: 157–160.

14 Marymont JH, Mills GQ, Merritt WD. Fracture of the lateral cuneiform bone in the absence of severe direct trauma. *American Journal of Sports Medicine* 1980; 8 (2): 135–136.

15 Creighton R, Sonogar A, Gordon G. Stress fracture of the tarsal middle cuneiform bone: a case report. *Journal of the American Podiatric Medical Association* 1990; 80: 489–495.

16 Khan KM, Brukner PD, Bradshaw C. Stress fracture of the medial cuneiform bone in a runner. *Clinical Journal of Sport Medicine* 1993; 3 (4): 262–264.

17 Khan KM, Brukner PD, Kearney C *et al*. Tarsal navicular stress fracture in athletes. *Sports Medicine* 1994; 17 (1): 65–76.

18 Waugh W. The ossification and vascularisation of the tarsal navicular and the relation to Kohler's disease. *Journal of Bone and Joint Surgery* 1958; 40B: 765–777.

19 Torg JS, Pavlov H, Cooley LH *et al*. Stress fractures of the tarsal navicular: a retrospective review of twenty-one cases. *Journal of Bone and Joint Surgery* 1982; 64-A: 700–712.

20 Fitch KD, Blackwell JB, Gilmour WN. Operation for non-union of stress fracture of the tarsal navicular. *Journal of Bone and Joint Surgery* 1989; 71B: 105–110.

21 Khan KM, Fuller PJ, Brukner PD, Kearney C, Burry HC. Outcome of conservative and surgical management of navicular stress fracture in athletes. *American Journal of Sports Medicine* 1992; 20: 657–666.

22 Matheson GO, Clement DB, McKenzie DC *et al*. Stress fractures in athletes: a study of 320 cases. *American Journal of Sports Medicine* 1987; 15: 46–58.

23 Benazzo F, Barnabei G, Ferrario A, Castelli C, Fischetto G. Stress fractures in track and field athletes. *Journal of Sports Traumatology and Related Research* 1992; 14: 51–65.

24 Brukner P, Bradshaw C, Khan K, White S. Stress fractures: a review of 180 cases. *Clinical Journal of Sport Medicine* 1996; 6 (2): 85–89.

25 Orava S, Karpakka J, Hulkko A, Takala T. Stress avulsion fracture of the tarsal navicular: an uncommon sports-related overuse injury. *American Journal of Sports Medicine* 1991; 19: 392–395.

26 Ting A, King W, Yocum L *et al*. Stress fractures of the tarsal navicular in long-distance runners. *Clinics in Sports Medicine* 1988; 7 (1): 89–101.

27 Hunter LY. Stress fracture of the tarsal navicular: more frequent than we realise? *American Journal of Sports Medicine* 1981; 9: 217–218.

28 Brukner P, Khan K. *Clinical Sports Medicine*. Sydney: McGraw Hill, 1993.

29 Pavlov H, Torg JS, Freiberger RH. Tarsal navicular stress fractures: radiographic evaluation. *Radiology* 1983; 148: 641–645.

30 Kiss ZA, Khan KM, Fuller PJ. Stress fractures of the tarsal navicular bone: CT findings in 55 cases. *American Journal of Roentgenology* 1993; 160: 111–115.

31 Orava S, Hulkko A. Delayed unions and nonunions of stress fractures in athletes. *American Journal of Sports Medicine* 1988; 16: 378–382.

32 Gordon TG, Solar J. Tarsal navicular stress fractures. *Journal of American Podiatric Medicine Association* 1985; 75: 363–366.

33 O'Connor K, Quirk R, Fricker P, Maguire K. Stress fracture of the tarsal navicular bone treated by bone grafting and internal fixation: three case studies and a literature review. *Excel* 1990; 6: 16–22.

34 Maitland GD. *Peripheral manipulation*. (3rd edn.) London: Butterworths, 1986.

35 Granter R. Soft tissue management of shin pain. (Abstract.) In: Australian Sports Medicine Federation, *Annual Conference in Sports Medicine*; 1993: 40.

36 Briethaupt MD. Fur pathologie des menschlichen fusses. *Medizinische Zeitung* 1855; 24: 169–177.

37 Harris RI, Beath T. The short first metatarsal: its incidence and clinical significance. *Journal of Bone and Joint Surgery* 1949; 31-A (3): 553–564.

38 Drez D, Young JC, Johnston RD, Parker WD. Metatarsal stress fractures. *American Journal of Sports Medicine* 1980; 8: 123–125.

39 Micheli LJ, Sohn RS, Soloman R. Stress fractures of the second metatarsal involving Lisfranc's joint in ballet dancers: a new overuse of the foot. *Journal of Bone and Joint Surgery* 1985; 67A: 1372–1375.

40 Harrington T, Crichton KJ, Anderson IF. Overuse ballet injury of the base of the second metatarsal. *American Journal of Sports Medicine* 1993; 21: 591–598.

41 O'Malley MJ, Hamilton WG, Munyak J, DeFranco MJ. Stress fractures at the base of the second metatarsal in ballet dancers. *Foot and Ankle International* 1996; 17 (2): 89–94.

42 Hamilton WG. Foot and ankle injuries in dancers. *Clinics in Sports Medicine* 1988; 7: 143–173.

43 Dameron TB. Fractures and anatomical variations of the proximal portion of the 5th metatarsal. *Journal of Bone and Joint Surgery* 1975; 57-A: 788–792.

44 Torg JS, Balduini FC, Zelko RR *et al*. Fractures of the base of the fifth metatarsal distal to the tuberosity: classification and guidelines for non-surgical and surgical management. *Journal of Bone and Joint Surgery* 1984; 66A: 209–214.

45 Richli WR, Rosenthal DJ. Avulsion fractures of the fifth metatarsal: experimental study of pathomechanics. *American Journal of Roentgenology* 1984; 143: 889–891.

46 Jones R. Fractures of the base of the 5th metatarsal bone by indirect violence. *Annals of Surgery* 1902; 34: 697–700.

47 Stewart IM. Jones' fractures: fracture of the base of the 5th metatarsal. *Clinical Orthopedic and Related Research* 1960; 16: 190–198.

48 Sammarco GJ. Be alert for Jones fractures. *Physician and Sportsmedicine* 1992; 20 (6): 101–109.

49 Shereff MJ, Yang QM, Kummer FJ *et al*. Vascular anatomy of the fifth metatarsal. *Foot and Ankle* 1991; 11 (6): 350–353.

50 Smith MJ, Arnoczky SP, Hersh A. The intraosseous blood supply of the fifth metatarsal: implications for proximal fracture healing. *Foot and Ankle* 1992; 13 (3): 143–152.

51 DeLee JC, Evans JP, Julian J. Stress fracture of the fifth metatarsal. *American Journal of Sports Medicine* 1983; 11: 349–353.

52 Clapper MF, O'Brien TJ, Lyons PM. Fractures of the fifth metatarsal: analysis of a fracture registry. *Clinical Orthopaedics and Related Research* 1995; 315: 239–241.

53 Mindrebo N, Shelbourne KD, Van Meter CD *et al*. Outpatient percutaneous screw fixation of the acute Jones fracture. *American Journal of Sports Medicine* 1993; 21 (5): 720–723.

54 Swanson SAV, Freeman MAR, Day WH. The fatigue properties of human cortical bone. *Medical and Biological Engineering* 1971; 9: 23–32.

55 Kavanaugh JH. The Jones fracture revisited. *Journal of Bone and Joint Surgery* 1978; 60-A: 776–782.

56 Zelko RR, Torg JS, Rachun A. Proximal diaphyseal fractures of the fifth metatarsal – treatment of the fractures and their complications in athletes. *American Journal of Sports Medicine* 1979; 7: 95–101.

57 Lawrence SR, Botte MJ. Jones' fracture and related fractures of the proximal fifth metatarsal. *Foot and Ankle* 1993; 14 (6): 358–365.

58 Helal B. The great toe sesamoid bones: the lus or lost souls of Ushaia. *Clinical Orthopaedics* 1981; 157: 82–87.

59 Van Hal ME, Keene JS, Lange TA, Clancy WGJ. Stress fractures of the great toe sesamoids. *American Journal of Sports Medicine* 1982; 10: 122–128.

60 Hulkko A, Orava S, Pellinen P, Puranen J. Stress fractures of the sesamoid bones of the first metatarsophalangeal joint in athletes. *Archives of Orthopaedic and Traumatic Surgery* 1985; 104: 113–117.

61 Inge GAL, Ferguson AB. Surgery of the sesamoid bones of the great toe. *Archives of Surgery* 1933; 27: 466–489.

62 Golding C. Museum pages V: the sesamoids of the hallux. *Journal of Bone and Joint Surgery* 1960; 42-B: 840–843.

63 Mann R. *DuVries Surgery of the Foot*. (4th edn.) St Louis: CV Mosby Co., 1978: 122–125.

64 Biedert R. Which investigations are required in stress fracture of the great toe sesamoids. *Journal of Orthopaedic and Trauma Surgery* 1993; 94–95.

65 Burton EM, Amaker BH. Stress fracture of the great toe sesamoid in a ballerina: MRI appearance. *Pediatric Radiology* 1994; 24: 37–38.

66 Davis AW, Alexander IJ. Problematic fractures and dislocations in the foot and ankle of athletes. *Clinics in Sports Medicine* 1990; 9: 163–181.

67 McBryde AM, Anderson RB. Sesamoid foot problems in the athlete. *Clinics in Sports Medicine* 1988; 7: 51–60.

68 Yokoe K, Mannoji T. Stress fracture of the proximal phalanx of the great toe: a report of three cases. *American Journal of Sports Medicine* 1986; 14 (3): 240–242.

69 Shiraishi M, Mizuta H, Kubota K, Sakuma K, Takagi K. Stress fracture of the proximal phalanx of the great toe. *Foot and Ankle* 1993; 14 (1): 28–34.

70 Gross TS, Bunch RP. A mechanical model of metatarsal stress fracture during distance running. *American Journal of Sports Medicine* 1989; 17: 669–674.

71 Mann RA, Hagy JL. The function of the toes in walking, jogging and running. *Clinical Orthopaedics* 1979; 142: 24–29.

72 Stokes IAF, Hutton WC, Stott JRR. Forces acting on the metatarsals during normal walking. *Journal of Anatomy* 1979; 129: 579–590.

73 Sammarco GJ. Biomechanics of the foot. In: Frankel VH, Nordin M, eds. *Basic Biomechanics of the Skeletal System*. Philadelphia: Lea and Febiger, 1980: 193–219.

74 Clanton TO, Butler JE, Eggert A. Injuries to metatarsophalangeal joint in athletes. *Foot and Ankle* 1986; 7: 162–176.

Index